Plant Based F
How to Improve Your Hea
Plant Ba
Copyright 20

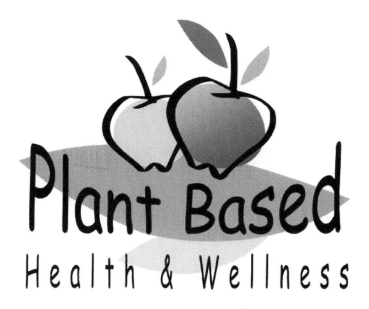

Preface

This is the story of my journey from obesity, heart disease, and Stage 3 kidney failure back to good health. I'll tell you right up front, I didn't do it perfectly, but even with several slips and setbacks, I stuck with the program and (eventually) made some amazing changes in my health.

I'm just an average person, who has lots of weaknesses and gives in to temptations easily, but I kept getting "back on the program" and that's how I eventually succeeded on the bumpy road to health.

Are you looking for an inspiring story that will lift you up and motivate you? This is that story. The simple program I describe in this book will change your life! I know that's a strong statement, but give me a chance to show you how it worked for me.

This approach is not about treating your symptoms; it's about getting to the root causes of disease and creating an environment in your body that will allow it to heal itself. Your body is an amazing self-healing machine!

Your body can heal itself if you give it a chance.
All you need to do is get rid of the toxins and provide it with healthy nutrients. This is a very simple approach to creating health!

Photo Gallery: The pictures that follow summarize my journey.

OK, this is embarrassing. Nobody wants to see his big fat belly hanging out, but I hope this photo gallery will convey the idea that change is possible.

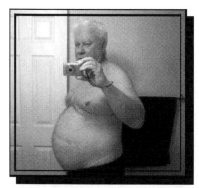

Weight 275 lbs, BP 228/137

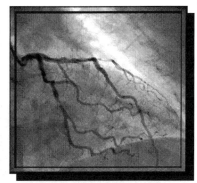

Clogged Arteries

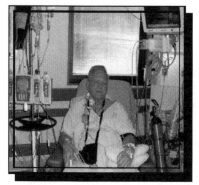

Open Heart Surgery

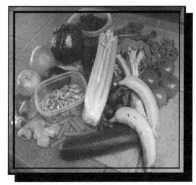

Healthy Plant-Based Diet

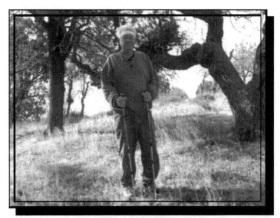

Hiking Again!

I want to stress that the program I describe in this book is not just about weight loss - it's about health. In fact, it's not just about health; it's about enjoying life and living with purpose!

Let's face it; if you live every day in pain, life is not that enjoyable. If you live with the fear that something awful is about to happen, life seems hardly worth the effort (I speak from experience). But if you live pain free, with hope for the future and a sense of purpose - now, that's an enjoyable life!

For me, weight loss was just a side benefit. Besides obesity, my health issues included heart attack and open heart surgery, dangerously high blood pressure, Stage 3 kidney failure, alcoholism, enlarged liver, neuropathy in my feet, a blood disorder (polycythemia vera), painful arthritis in my shoulders, numbness in my left arm, and partial blindness in my right eye. OK, I was a sick puppy.

I felt like I was standing on the edge of a cliff, and was about to fall over. What a precarious situation! Instead of that, I was able to back away from the edge and put some distance between myself and disaster.

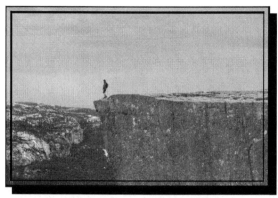

Standing on the Edge

If I'm not an expert, how can I presume to write a book like this? Well, we're talking about my life. I lived this story and learned a few things along the way that I would like to share with you. My pain was real, and my healing was real.

Here's how it all started.

November 29, 2017, Emergency Room at the VA Medical Center

"I woke up this morning with my left arm completely numb. Not like when you sleep on it wrong, this numbness didn't go away. Also, I was partially blind in my right eye. There was a big black spot obscuring part of the visual field. I thought I had a stroke. So, after getting cleaned up I went directly to the emergency room at the VA medical center.

I am obese with extremely high blood pressure, but I thought little of it because I drink a 12-pack of beer every day and just kind of hope nothing bad would happen. Boy, was I wrong!

Is this really me? When I was young I could do anything and get away with it. Now, at 73, I have:

1. *Dangerously high blood pressure at 228/137.*
2. *Left arm has gone numb.*
3. *Partial blindness in right eye.*
4. *With a hematocrit (HCT) of 57.2% the oncologists said that my blood chemistry indicates I have bone marrow cancer (polycythemia vera).*
5. *A CAT scan showed that I have an enlarged liver.*
6. *With an eGFR of 38 mL/min, I am in Stage-3 kidney failure. My primary care physician said the next thing is dialysis and then death. (We'll talk more about interpreting your blood test results in Appendix E).*
7. *Itching, rashes and sores all over my body.*

8. *Ocular migraines.*

9. *The neuropathy in my feet causes my legs to jerk at night, so I can't sleep very well. Also, the arthritis in my shoulders makes it so I can only lie on my side for a short while. Therefore I flop back and forth all night just waiting for it to be morning. Right now I dread going to bed. This has to change!*

10. *Because of my excess weight I have trouble walking. I struggle just to walk from the bedroom to the living room without holding on to everything in sight. At the grocery store I use the shopping cart as a walker. I haven't resorted to using their little electric carts, but that's the next step. Also, I find it difficult just to bend over and pick up something off the floor. I used to be a strong hiker, now look at me!*

11. *The chest X-ray showed a spot on my lungs.*

12. *The emergency room doctor said I have too much blood and wants to take some off. What! Bloodletting? I thought they did away with that during the Middle Ages!*

13. *Am I going to become disabled or die from a stroke?*

I have some serious health issues, and need to make some major changes. Hopefully it is not too late."

Why another book on health and lifestyle changes? Aren't there enough of them already? Why do I feel compelled to share my story?

Well, maybe something you find here will resonate with your unique situation. Maybe there is something that I share, that will strike a responsive chord.

If you are motivated to make some changes and improve your health by something you find in this book, I will be overjoyed!

So, here's some straight talk. If you are overweight and have high blood pressure, it is LIKELY that you will have a heart attack or a stroke. I'm not trying to use a scare tactic; I'm just telling you the way it is. You may be thinking, "It won't happen to me" but I'm telling you this because I've been there. It can, and probably will, happen to you!

Take action now to avoid some of the things I have lived through. For half of all heart attack victims the first symptom is death. In other words, they don't get any early warning signs; they just suffer a massive heart attack and die. Then it's too late to make any diet or lifestyle changes; they are already dead.

I'm not talking about life and death. We're all going to die. Hopefully that doesn't come as a surprise to you.

What I am talking about is **quality of life** while you are still alive.
If you live a long and healthy life and then go down quickly at the end, that's a good thing. It's called "compression of morbidity."

Do you want to finish out your life partially paralyzed, blind, or suffering with severe chest pains? We're talking serious stuff here! If you follow the plan described in this book, you may avoid some of the dreadful things I have had to endure. When you have allergic reactions to all of your blood pressure medications (tongue and throat swelling), it's scary and painful!

Even if you already have some serious health issues, it may not be too late. You may be able to slow their progress or even reverse these issues by making a few simple diet and lifestyle changes! I did.

The Standard American Diet (SAD) that consists of processed foods loaded with fat, salt, sugar, and toxic chemicals causes obesity, diabetes, high blood pressure, heart disease, and cancer. If you wanted to design a diet that would cause disease, you couldn't do better than the Standard American Diet.

> Fast foods and prepackaged meals taste great, but they will kill you!

It has been shown in several well-documented studies that diabetes, heart disease, and even dementia (type 3 diabetes) can be prevented and even reversed. You may think that is an outrageous claim. If so, I urge you to watch the video documentaries and read the books listed in Appendix A. These resources demonstrate this principle very clearly.

Given a chance, the human body is an amazing self-healing machine. In fact, your body is healing right now, and it works all the time, 24 hours a day! If it didn't, you would die in a short period of time. Sometimes the healing process is obvious like when you cut your finger, but most of the internal healing and immune system functions we are completely unaware of.

The plan I am proposing is not a juice fast; it's a long term, sustainable, plant-based way of eating combined with mild exercise. Also, if you are like me, you don't have the money to attend fancy health and wellness retreats or check into a rehab center. This is a program you can do on your own without spending lots of money. Following the simple steps described in this book has completely changed my life, both physically and emotionally, and it will change your life too!

How do you make changes regarding habits you have been practicing for a lifetime? How do you make these changes if you are like me and have no willpower?

I had a heart attack and triple bypass open-heart surgery eight years ago and even that wasn't enough to scare me into permanent lifestyle change. It was enough for a few short-term changes, but after a few months I was right back to my old ways, drinking a 12-pack of beer every day and eating loads of junk food.

Different people are motivated in different ways. Fear and sickness were not enough for me. Willpower and toughing it out were not enough for me. The secret for me this time around was to get excited about making these changes and to ENJOY THE JOURNEY, not struggle with it.

This program represents a change of mindset - a different way of looking at life. Willpower and toughing it out won't last very long, but joy and hope are wonderful motivators that are sustainable. Also, once you have reclaimed your health, you will want to help others on their way to health. The joy of helping others will last the rest of your life!

I consider this program as a gift to an undeserving person - me. I'm telling you, if I can start at 73 years old as an obese, sick, alcoholic, and completely change my life (even though I had MANY false starts and setbacks) you can too! It's NOT too late!

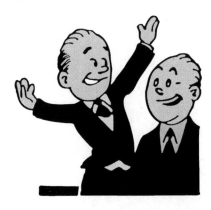

So, what's the key to success? For me it was twelve fold:

1. **Sobriety**: I couldn't follow any health program when I was drinking. I could talk a good story, but couldn't put it into action.
2. **Healthy Eating**: Whole foods, plant based.
3. **Mild Exercise**: For me it is hiking.
4. **A Positive Expectation**: I believed from the beginning (without a doubt) that this program would work and I would achieve my goals. I learned along the way that setbacks are only temporary. In fact setbacks are part of the learning process and make you stronger.
5. **Educating Myself**: I learned about nutrition and health by watching documentaries and reading books.
6. **Embracing the Effort**: I had to recognize and embrace the idea that it was going to take some effort. I learned to view the hard or boring parts as just part of the process.

7. **Emotional Involvement**: Intellect alone doesn't do it. Emotional involvement drives these lessons deep into your being.
8. **Stress Management**: For me stress management consists of relaxation, visualization, and prayer.
9. **Staying away from the edge.** I can't flirt with temptation and get away with it. If I think about some unhealthy behavior long enough, I'll end up doing it. So, I have to plot a course that keeps me far away from the edge.
10. **Learning to Treat Myself as if I Mattered:** This was a tough lesson for me because my feelings of inferiority were part of my personality, but people can change.
11. **Gratitude**: No matter what your religious beliefs, you probably believe in some kind of Higher Power. I wake up each morning grateful for the opportunity to live another day, and that sets the tone for the entire day.
12. **Share Your Journey**: Try to help others get motivated and get healthy. Trying to help others (without being obnoxious) is very motivating to me, and is part of "Love your neighbor as yourself."

Frankly, if you are not an alcoholic you are WAY ahead of the game. Getting off the beer is the hardest thing I've ever done. Drinking a 12-pack of beer each day absolutely prevented me from living a healthy lifestyle. Over the past several years I learned a lot of things about health, and I have thought a lot about health, but I didn't do anything about it. Only after I got sober was I able to start making healthy choices.

If you have a food addiction, that's pretty similar to alcoholism. It's a big strike against you, but I believe the principles described in this book will help you overcome it.

Following the few simple lifestyle changes described here I have accomplished the following:

1. I brought my blood pressure down to normal, and don't need to take any prescription medications (and don't have to worry about allergic reactions).
2. I lost 50 pounds.
3. The neuropathy in my feet, and the arthritis in my shoulders are almost gone.
4. I can walk and even do strenuous hikes without any pain in my legs.
5. My blood work is normal with no indication of kidney failure or cancer.
6. I discovered a greater purpose for living.

I was able to achieve all this with just a few simple diet and lifestyle changes. Talk about a miracle drug! There were no drugs involved. In fact, another theme of this book is to get off all prescription drugs as soon as possible.

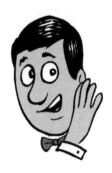

Tips and Tricks

When you see this little guy, you know he is offering some interesting tips to make your life easier or just a silly comment to lighten things up.

What I thought I could accomplish in six months actually took over a year because of my slips and false starts, but getting back on the program right away instead of getting discouraged and quitting eventually paid off!

Thanks:

I would like to thank two people who have been very helpful as I traveled along this bumpy road.

Tim McGee. Tim is my primary care physician at the VA Medical Center. His genuine concern and encouragement were very motivating, and helped me stay on track.

Gerard Coard. Gerard has given me many great suggestions and a lot of encouragement. In fact, a few of his inspiring comments appear in the Diary section of Chapter 4.

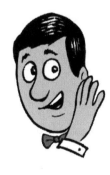

"Stories of amazing life-changing recoveries usually come from 'young people' in their 40s and 50s, but at this writing, I am 75 years old, and I'm telling you that you can do this!
Give it a try. You will completely change your life and the lives of those around you!"

If you enjoy this book, please leave a nice 5-Star review on amazon.com. It will help spread the word.

OK, let's get started!

Table of Contents

Chapter 1. I'm in Big Trouble!

Chapter 2. The Lowdown on Foods

Chapter 3. Foods, Spices, and Gadgets

Chapter 4. How Am I Doing?

Chapter 5. Wow! Emotional Healing Too?

Chapter 6. The "E" Word

Chapter 7. My "Big Adventure"

Chapter 8. Fifteen Months Later

Chapter 1. I'm in Big Trouble!

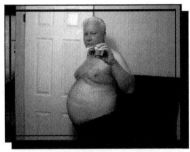

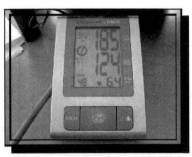

Weight 275 Pounds   Blood Pressure 185/124

1.1 A Wakeup Call

I had a heart attack and triple bypass open-heart surgery eight years ago. It was a huge event in my life, and you would think that would have been enough to motivate me to permanent change! Well, not true.

I made a bunch of lifestyle changes that lasted only a few months, and then it was back to my old ways. I was drinking a 12-pack of beer every day and eating loads of junk food. What's the definition of stupid?

1.1.1 Eight Years Later

So now, eight years later I am obese, have super high blood pressure (185/124) and am in serious trouble. A month ago I ended up in the emergency room with blood pressure of 228/137 and my left arm had gone numb. Was it a stroke? Probably.

I don't want to end up permanently disabled because of a major stroke or struggling for years with frightening chest pains. When I have chest pains I always wonder, "Am I going to drop dead right now?" That's a scary feeling! Who wants to have their feet amputated, go blind, or be hooked up to a dialysis machine? Those are very real possibilities for me. Instead I would like to get back to hiking, treasure hunting, and shooting nature photographs.

What will it take for me to make permanent change? If you are reading this book, it's been long enough for me to have made the necessary changes and achieve some major successes. Otherwise this book would never have been completed.

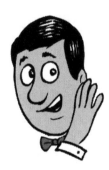

"Most people do nothing about their health until they end up with some serious problems. You don't need to wait that long!"

So, I've had another wake up call, and I have learned some valuable lessons that I want to share with you. Maybe you can learn from my experiences and not have to go through them yourself!

1.2 Where Will I Be in a Year?

1.2.1 My Goal List

In a year from starting this program I hope to have achieved the following:

1. Healthy weight.
2. Strength enough to enjoy hiking and other outdoor activities.
3. Eliminate the neuropathy in my feet.
4. Eliminate the arthritis in my shoulders.
5. Normal blood pressure without prescription drugs

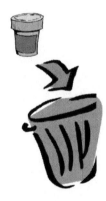

1.3 Effective Motivation Is the Key!

This may be the most important section in this book. If you can stay motivated, you can accomplish anything. If not, you'll accomplish nothing! Sheer willpower and "toughing it out" won't last long. You have to stay motivated and excited about the journey you have started.

> The things I mention in this section are not just some cute sayings from a self-help book. These are the powerful principles that I needed to use in order to make huge and lasting changes in my life.

1.3.1 Become Emotionally Involved

I knew I was in deep trouble with my health. When I would watch a documentary about people who were getting well, I would weep. These stories touched something deep within me. I'm not a psychologist, but I think emotional involvement can help motivate you at a deep level. Treating your health program as a purely intellectual endeavor will guarantee failure.

Of course, positive emotions like joy and hope are much better motivators than anger, fear, and beating yourself up. The concept of emotional involvement permeates all of the other keys that I will mention in this section.

I have always been a pretty stoic, unemotional person. An engineer by trade, I looked at life logically, and approached projects in a matter of fact way. Now that my life is on the line, that approach isn't going to work!

When you picture yourself healthy, feel the emotions that come with a thin, strong body. Feel the joy that comes with freedom - freedom from pain and anxiety. These feelings are a strong motivator for success.

1.3.2 Positive vs. Negative Motivation

I have very little willpower and I'm not just being modest when I say that; It's a fact. I'm always amazed at people who say they are going to do something and then they just go ahead and do it. So what takes the place of willpower for me?

Passion!

In recent years I have become a pretty emotional person, and I can get passionate about things. The little bit of progress I achieved during the first week of this program was so exciting and motivating! Now, a month into it, I am very passionate and FILLED with excitement and joy. I think about my goals and the progress I'm making all the time! The motivation is positive, not negative. It's based more on joy than fear. The only things you need to give up are those things that are bad for you, and the things you acquire are all good for you.

Can I keep up this level of excitement? Well, that's what the rest of the points in this Section are about.

1.3.3 Jump in with Both Feet!

Jumping in with both feet makes an adventure out of it and emphasizes the fact that this is a MAJOR LIFE CHANGE with no going back! It's a way of making a commitment and sticking with it.

"Moderation in all things" doesn't work for most people. It certainly doesn't work for me. Instead of teasing myself by eating some unhealthy foods and thinking that I'll gradually migrate over to a healthy diet, I decided to make a clean break. That's the simple way to go. There are no complicated decisions to make, so for me it was much easier. You may feel differently, but for me this program is all encompassing. I'm sure my alcohol addiction was part of that decision. I quit drinking altogether. Again, moderate drinking is not an option for me.

Eating some junk food just reminds me how much I like it. Jumping in 100% will allow my taste buds to change much quicker. Believe it or not, after only a few weeks I started to crave vegetable juice with lots of kale and cabbage. Of course, a little fruit helps to sweeten it up, especially a little bit of lemon. Eating a variety of colors and tastes is important.

Undoubtedly there are some few people who can find moderation, but the vast majority of us just can't. So, I gave up all animal products and manufactured foods completely.

1.3.4 The Healthy Cycle

You have heard about "The Viscous Cycle" or "The Downward Spiral." Well, how about "The Healthy Cycle?"

As pictured in Figure 3-1, when you loose weight you will feel like being more active, and as you become more active you will loose more weight. Enjoying the progress you have made motivates you toward more progress. Of course, this program is not just about loosing weight; it's about getting healthy!

27

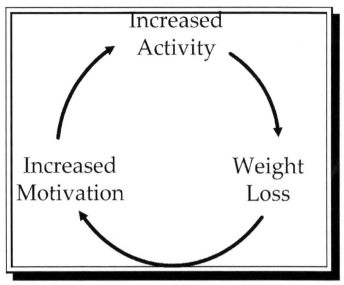

Figure 3-1 The Healthy Cycle

1.3.5 Have a Plan with Specific Goals

Think about where you are right now and where you want to be in a month or a year. Having a plan with specific goals is motivating, and it's the best way to ensure that you are on track. It's best if you write it down and look at it every so often.

Writing your goals down makes them more concrete and increases the likelihood of you achieving them.

If the captain of a cargo ship just left the harbor with no idea of where he was going or how to get there, where would he end up? Who knows, maybe on some desert island or maybe right back where he started. The same idea applies to your health program. If you have specific goals and make course corrections along the way, you will reach those goals.

Also, break really big goals down into several smaller ones. Your big goals may seem so huge that you get discouraged. For example, when I started this program I weighed 275 pounds. I knew that I needed to reach 225 pounds at least. Loosing 50 pounds seemed overwhelming! I was so far away from that!

So, I didn't worry about loosing 50 pounds. I set five pound goals. When I reached 270 pounds that was a great accomplishment, and I started to focus on 265 pounds. Of course, I wanted to reach my 225-pound goal as quickly as possible, but I took it a little at a time and eventually reached it! When things seemed to be progressing too slowly, I had to remind myself, "This is a lifelong journey. Just keep on keeping on and you will get there."

Each time I saw my primary care physician I wanted to show a lot of progress since the last visit. Is that vanity? Maybe, but it was a motivator for me!

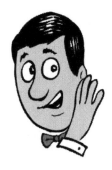

"Make sure your goals are:
1. Specific
2. Measurable
3. Realistic"

1.3.6 Keep Track of Your Progress

If you are a nerd like me you already like to keep track of stuff, but if not you will still be motivated by seeing your progress summarized in a table or in a diary. This morning the scales revealed that I had lost another pound. I couldn't wait to record it in my BP/Weight log.

Day by day you may not notice your gains, but when you summarize them for a month - wow! It's amazing.

What to keep track of? I'm sure you will find other things to track. Here are a few of mine:

1. Blood pressure
2. Weight
3. Progress on my baseline hike
4. Health diary

I record my blood pressure and weight each day, but I make entries in the diary only every so often. Seeing progress in your BP/Weight log can be very motivating, but it will also point out very clearly what happens when you get off track. It's then that you need to recommit to the program.

This is one of the most motivational things that I do. I watch health and wellness documentaries on FMTV almost every day. It pumps me up like crazy. I love seeing real life stories about people who have made a few simple changes and have accomplished amazing feats of healing in their lives.

Also, in some of these videos you get to see the awful side of industrial farming and food manufacturing. You see how they treat the animals (hard to watch), and how food manufacturers introduce toxins and chemicals into their highly processed and packaged foods. There is a subscription fee for FMTV (about the same as Netflix). You may think it is too expensive, but ask yourself what your health is worth. How much does a heart attack or a stroke cost? I speak from experience. Fortunately I am regaining strength in my left arm and the vision in my right eye is returning. You don't need to get in as bad a shape as I did before making some healthy changes! Even if you are already dealing with some serious health issues, it's not too late. The body wants to heal its self. We just need to create an environment where it can.

This may sound corny but:

1. A foolish man doesn't learn from his mistakes.
2. A smart man does learn from his mistakes.
3. A wise man learns from the mistakes of others.

Today we are fortunate because there are literally hundreds of educational and motivational videos available. As more people are becoming aware, there are new videos being introduced almost every day. Also, there are many wonderful, easy to understand books available. A quick search on YouTube will provide lots of interesting videos on almost every topic relating to health and wellness. We have a wealth of information available to us!

1.3.8 Plan for a "Big Adventure"

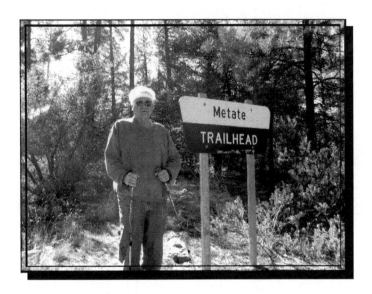

If you plan for a major event and then achieve it, that will give your motivation a huge boost! Your "big adventure" should be something that you couldn't do at the beginning of your health journey, but you know is achievable. Maybe you want to run a marathon or climb a mountain. Maybe you want to get out of your wheelchair and walk around the block. It all depends on where you are starting from and where you want to be. Of course, once you achieve that goal you can go on to greater things.

For me it was a hike up to Blair Pass on Granite Mountain. Now, for healthy people in good shape a 3.2-mile hike might not seem like a big deal, but only a few months ago I could barely walk! So for me, it was a big deal - a really big deal. Now that I have done that, I'm setting my sights on a hike up to the summit of Granite Mountain. I'm starting to learn that most of our limitations are self-imposed.

1.3.9 Enjoy Every Victory, Even the Small Ones

Here's a perfect example. This is my diary entry for January 2, 2018.

"Today I 'broke into' the 240's. When I saw 249 on the scale I was very pleased. I started this journey at 275 pounds and have a goal of getting down to 225 pounds, so I still have a long way to go. But this is an exciting milestone. I'm really enjoying this small victory!"

1.3.10 Look Back Down the Mountain

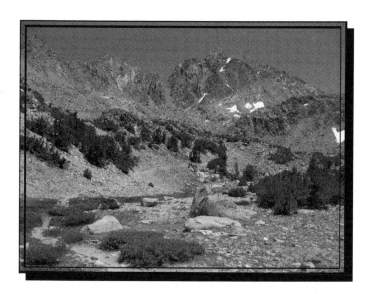

I used to do a lot of backpacking in the Sierra Nevada Mountains of California. Almost every day we would have to climb a long and steep trail to reach a high mountain pass.

Instead of always looking up toward the pass (which just didn't seem to be getting any closer) I would periodically look back down the mountain and see how far I had come. I knew that just putting one foot in front of the other would eventually get me there. And, sure enough, before you know it I was on the top!

This same approach can keep you motivated to keep making progress toward a far off goal.

Instead of always focusing on how far you have to go, look back on how much you have already accomplished. If you focus too much on your long-term goals, they can seem so big and far away that you will get discouraged and quit. Focusing on your accomplishments will motivate you to keep moving forward.

Don't worry so much about your eventual goal; you WILL get there. Just enjoy the journey all along the way. If you "keep on keeping on" you will reach that goal before you know it. So, every once in a while look back down the mountain.

1.3.11 Stay in Touch with Supportive Friends

I have always been a loner. I am single, live alone, and don't answer to anybody. I don't like the idea of joining support groups and all that kind of stuff (including AA). But I have learned that it is important to have some kind of "support group" or "community" even if it is just one friend who you keep in touch with via email. This way you will have someone who you can share ideas with and you can encourage each other. Being accountable to someone is a great step toward success. I have a friend who lives in a different city. We never see each other, but we exchange emails a couple of times each week. This has proven to be a great help to me (and hopefully to him) for staying motivated, and staying on track. So, if you are alone, don't give up hope. I'm sure you have at least one friend with whom you can share things.

Your support group might even be an online community or forum. Some of my favorites include iThrive, FMTV, and Reboot with Joe. A quick search of the Internet for "health and wellness forums" will yield several excellent forums. Also, there are lots of health and wellness groups on Facebook. The members of these groups are going through the same things that you are, and they are very encouraging. Not only are they supportive, they can be a wealth of helpful experience-based information.

1.3.12 Visualize Your Success

I'll talk in more detail about this topic later, but for now let me just say that picturing yourself as having already achieved your goals is a strong motivator. In Section 1.8.7, I describe a specific technique that I use, but you can picture yourself as you want to be any time, anywhere just by holding the image in your mind. Also, it's important to include emotion with your visualization. Imagine what it will feel like when you reach your goal.

Besides having a relaxation/visualization session each day I have put up a "vision board" in my bedroom. It is the first thing I see when I wake up each morning.

A vision board is just a bulletin board where you post pictures of the things you want to accomplish. It might contain:

1. Pictures of you when you were in better shape. If you don't have any pictures like that cut out a picture of someone who is in great shape and paste your face on it.
2. A vacation or retreat you would like to take.
3. The home you would like to own.
4. The amount of money you would like to have in your bank account.
5. The soul mate you hope to find when you are lean and sexy.

Don't be "realistic" or limit your dreams. Think big! Right now I am just about broke, but I still put up a picture of my dream home with a beautiful library and a $100,000.00 bill (OK, it's a $1.00 bill, but I wrote $100,000.00 on it). I also have a picture of me when I was young and strong. Can I be that way again? Well, I sure can be a lot closer than I am right now! Figure 1-2 is a picture of my vision board.

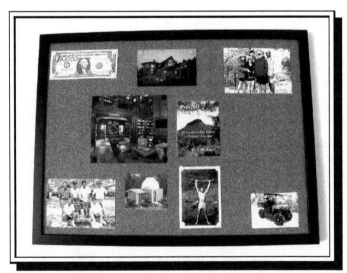

Figure 1-2 My Vision Board

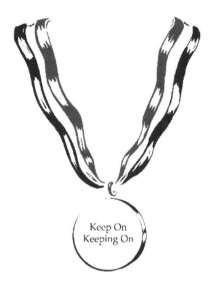

It seems like nothing in life is linear. We don't travel in a straight line from where we are to our goals. We almost always travel in "fits and starts" with plateaus along the way. Sometimes we may actually take a few steps backwards. That's OK. Don't sweat it! I had MANY slips and setbacks on this journey, but I consider them all part of the learning process.

If you keep track of your weight every day, you will see that it can vary up or down somewhat depending on how much water you retain or if you had a bad night's sleep. If you are consistently living a healthy life style, the overall trend will be toward your ideal weight.

My scale is digital and only displays whole numbers. So, if the scale reads 242 lbs, my actual weight might be 241.5. It will read 241 eventually.

Slips are a different story. Over the course of this journey I had several slips regarding my beer drinking, and boy did I pay the price - emotionally and physically! One night I simply decided that I was going to have some beer. I drank a 12-pack and ate an entire pizza. I knew better, but just decided that that's what I wanted to do. The next morning my weight and blood pressure had jumped dramatically and I felt disappointed in myself. It took a week to get back to where I was before the slip, but the important thing is that I didn't give up and quit altogether.

The lesson for me was to realize that the alcoholic within me doesn't go away or sleep. He is just waiting for me to relax a little bit and then he comes charging back with a vengeance! If I allowed it, he would take me right back to where I was very quickly. Your demon may be sugar, tobacco, or junk food, but the lesson is still the same. Once you know the enemy you can be alert and vigilant.

I'm not encouraging you to get off track, but I can almost guarantee that you will. We each need to realize that we are only human beings just doing the best we can. I would like to think that I am stronger than I am, but I'm just an average guy.

So, what do you do if you slip? Just get back on the program immediately. Don't beat yourself up. In fact, don't even worry about it. It's not the end of the world, and it's certainly not the end of your healthy living program. It's only the end when you give up and quit. Forget your setbacks and just keep on keeping on.

This program is about progress, not perfection. It's better to be a little bit patient with yourself, have a few slips, and get right back on the program than it is to be a rigid perfectionist. If you are too rigid and insist on perfection, you will probably give up in discouragement and quit. Then it really is over!

Which of the two graphs below would you like to describe your progress? Figure 1-3 shows a rough and rocky road with some setbacks, but the overall progress is upward. Figure 1-4 starts out gangbusters, but this person is rigid and inflexible with an all-or-nothing approach. When things don't happen exactly the way he thinks they should he is ready to throw in the towel.

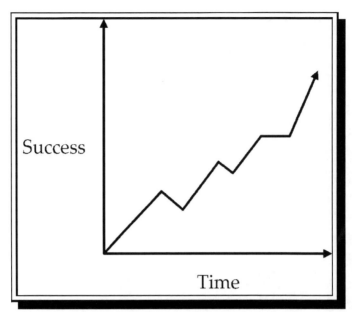

Figure 1-3 The Rocky Road to Success

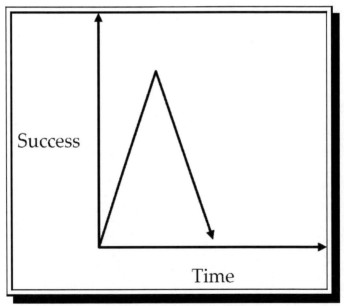

Figure 1-4 The Smooth Road to Failure

Now, this program is not just about weight loss, but weight loss is a good indicator of your progress. The most important numbers are blood pressure and blood chemistry. You can't have your blood labs done every day, but you can weigh yourself every day.

I started this journey at 275 pounds. When I had reached 235 pounds I got off track big time. I spent a week eating packaged foods and drinking beer. I thought to myself, "I can't do this. It's just too hard!" Then I had to remind myself, "Hey, you have lost 40 pounds and your blood pressure is starting to come down. That's amazing progress! Don't quit now; just get back on the program and do the best you can. You will succeed at this!" I had to look back down the mountain.

When I think back on some of these things I don't beat myself up, in fact I have great compassion on myself realizing how weak and pathetic I am. I'm 75 years old, but often I feel like a child trying to please his demanding parents. I'm just doing the best I can. My best may not be very good, but it is good enough for success.

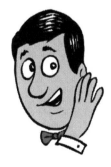

"There is no such thing as failure. You just haven't reached your goal yet. The only way for you to fail is if you quit altogether."

Think of a beautiful mountain stream like the one shown in Figure 1-5. There may be rocks or other obstacles along the way, but the water finds a way around them. It's the same for your health journey. Maybe there are some obstacles in your path, but you can find a way around them!

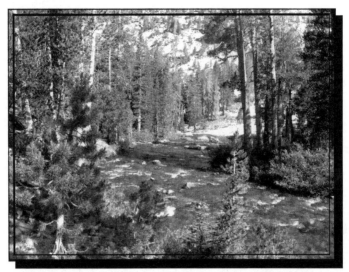

Figure 1-5 Think of a Mountain Stream

1.3.14 Stay Away From the Edge

This may seem a little technical, but hopefully some may like the illustration. As shown in Figure 1-6 our simple yes/no decisions (Am I going to break down and eat that junk food?) can be pictured as a cusp surface.

Path "A" stays well away from the danger zone near the edge, but path "B" travels close to the cusp. It won't take much of a pull by influence X to pull Path B it over the edge. In other words, stay well away from temptation. If you don't want to eat junk food, don't buy it and bring it into your home. Be smart and don't go shopping hungry. Have something to eat before heading out to the grocery store.

Your addiction may be sugar, cigarettes, alcohol, or cocaine. People who are not alcoholics or food addicts honestly don't understand the pleasure of the addiction or the powerful pull that it has. My greatest addiction is to alcohol. When I am immersed in this healthy living program I am occupied with thoughts of:

1. Wow! My weight is dropping!
2. My blood pressure is coming down, and will soon be normal without taking any drugs.
3. My odds of having a stroke or becoming diabetic are decreasing.
4. I don't have to worry about having an allergic reaction to my blood pressure medicine.
5. My vision is improving and I probably won't go blind.
6. I wake up feeling refreshed and wanting to get up and pursue some interesting projects.
7. The neuropathy in my feet is almost gone.
8. I'm starting to be able to move without pain.
9. My last checkup was great! All of my blood and urine numbers are coming into the normal range.
10. I have saved a lot of money by not buying a 12-pack of beer each day.
11. I feel great and have hope for the future!

When I forget all these things and stray too close to the edge I start to think:

1. It would be fun to drink some beer and eat junk food tonight. If I allow myself to start thinking about it very long, I'll do it!

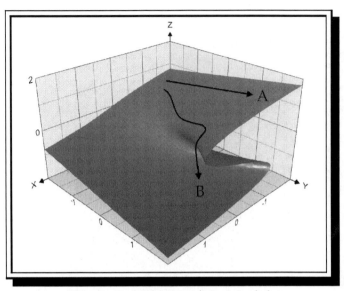

Figure 1-6 The Yes/No Model

This is probably the hardest one for me. I'm not sure where it came from, but I have always had an inferiority complex and thought of myself as less important than others. When something bad would happen in my life, I usually thought that I deserved it because it was the result of something I did wrong.

I don't think that I have completely recovered from my insecurities, but today I believe that I do have some worth and that I should treat myself with respect. Think of a friend that you love and admire. How would you treat that person? Well, that's how I am trying to treat myself.

One of my favorite hobbies is treasure hunting. I love to go out with my metal detector to old mining sites and abandoned homesteads. It's exciting to find an old coin or a piece of jewelry, but think about what a treasure your health is!

I have already been in the position where I could barely walk because of the pain in my legs, and could hardly sleep at night because my legs would unexpectedly jump from the neuropathy in my feet (my legs feel completely out of control). The arthritis in my shoulders made it so that I could only sleep about a half-hour at a time. I would toss and turn all night just watching the clock and waiting for the night to be over. Also, the pain in my right shoulder is so bad that if I want to raise my right arm above my head I have to assist it with the other arm (some of you may know what that's like).

I have already experienced partial blindness in my right eye, allergic reactions to blood pressure medications, and chest pains that made me wonder, "Am I going to die right now?" If you are at peace with your Creator the thought of dying isn't that scary, but when it becomes an immediate reality you would rather have some options.

Think about these conditions only getting worse. Where does that lead? It leads to more immobility, more pain, blindness, and who knows what else! Now, what would it be like to discover perfect health? What kind of treasure would that be to find?

When I compare my health to a hidden treasure it is very motivating to me. But, I have to realize that I won't find it hidden under a rock somewhere; I can only reclaim my health by consistently working the program described in this book. Even if you have never been out treasure hunting, thinking about your health as a hidden treasure is a great motivator.

1.3.17 Have A Sense of Purpose

That awful day in the emergency room was a change point for me. Instead of thinking, "I'm in an awful situation, so I'll just have to deal with it and do the best I can" I started thinking, "Maybe I can use my experience to help others." This approach gave a sense of purpose to my life and is one of the most motivating factors for my success. Now it's not just me feeling sorry for myself; it's me seeking to help other people.

It seems to be the case that transformation is often preceded by crisis. If you study people who are living a life filled with purpose, you will usually find they had some experience that prompted them to action. Many drug abuse counselors were once addicts themselves. Many health and wellness advocates have suffered severe health issues - either themselves or a loved one. These things gave them experience in their chosen field, and also their desire to use those experiences to help others added purpose and meaning to their lives.

Sharing my health journey with you by writing this book has added purpose to my life. Hopefully you can use your journey to help others. If we all encourage each other toward success, the world will be a better place!

When I finally publish this book, is my purpose fulfilled and over? No, it will have just begun! Going through my own health journey and writing this book marked a change point in my life. Getting away from my life-long habit of excessive alcohol consumption and eating junk food marks the beginning of a new phase of my life. Learning about the joy of encouraging and motivating others on their health journey also marks the beginning of a life-long purpose for me. I'm already 75 years old, but because of the diet and lifestyle changes I have made, I look forward to many more purpose-filled years.

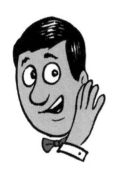

"When I first heard about this plant-based lifestyle I was very excited! I wanted to share it with everyone, but nobody was interested. Why? Because I hadn't shown any progress myself. Once people started to see the dramatic progress I was making, they became interested and started making changes of their own. I didn't have to preach or twist arms, they were motivated by seeing my progress!"

If you have a sense of purpose, you will have a reason to get out of bed in the morning. Your purpose is your reason to live. Life will be more interesting and exciting, and it will improve your health.

If you don't know what your purpose is, think back over your life and ask yourself:

1. What things have brought me joy in the past?
2. What am I good at? What special talents do I have?
3. What things do I like to do?
4. What ideas am I passionate about?
5. What endeavors have I been most successful at?
6. What things have people complemented me on?
7. Given the opportunity, what would I like to devote my whole energy to?

Your interests, talents, and successes are a clue as to what you are suited for. Discover your purpose and start living it!

1.3.18 Start Each Day With Gratitude

Each morning before I get out of bed I just lay there for a few minutes thinking how thankful I am for my improving health and how amazing it is to live another day. I think about what I hope to accomplish that day and am grateful for the opportunity to try and accomplish those things. If you are a religious person, this is a good time for a short prayer. I give thanks for a new day and pray that I will think and act in such a way that God will be pleased. This is very motivating for me and sets the tone for the whole day.

1.4 In Just One Month!

Section 4.3 has some excerpts from my Health Diary. There you can track my progress over time, but let me just share one entry with you right now. This entry shows you how motivating even a small success can be.

January 1, 2018, Happy New Year!

"December 2017 was a good month. I lost 25 pounds, and my blood pressure went from extremely high to normal (still taking BP meds). I am regaining strength in my left arm, and the vision in my right eye is almost back to normal. The pain in my legs is gone, so I am back to regular hiking. The congestion and coughing fits are gone. I'm sleeping much better and getting up earlier. I feel much more energetic and am spending more time on my various projects (including this book). I saved about $400 by not buying a 12-pack of beer every day. All that in one month! Wow, this program is working!"

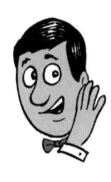

"With a fast start like that, I thought I would reach my health goals in six months. Well, it didn't go exactly that way. With my false starts and setbacks, it took over a year. But, the important thing is that I didn't give up and quit. After each setback, I got right back on the program and did eventually reach my goals! Because everything didn't go smoothly I am in a better position for permanent change.
I tell you this up front, because you will probably run into some tough spots along the way too. Don't give up; just keep on keeping on!"

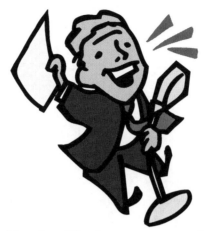

Here's a Big Announcement!

Treating symptoms is not addressing the underlying condition! Take a good hard look at the picture below. Which of these options do you want? You don't have to be Albert Einstein to know that the pharmaceutical approach only treats symptoms (with devastating side effects) and the nutritional approach will boost your immune system and only have positive side effects. You were meant to be healthy, so give your body a chance!

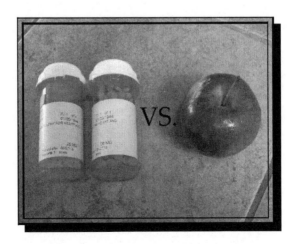

There is a paradigm shift happening in America right now in 2018! Are you aware of it? Millions of people; doctors, insurance companies, and patients are asking, "Why just treat the symptoms of disease when we can treat the root cause and get well?"

This is a completely different paradigm!
It's the difference is between disease management and health creation.
All chronic diseases can be prevented or reversed. You may have had a chronic disease for years. Why put up with that? It can be reversed or cured in a mater of weeks or months! Think about it;
This idea will bring about a whole new era in health care in America and around the world. This is the future of medicine, and it is coming just in time to prevent our medical system from going bankrupt.

Promoting health and avoiding disease is much more cost effective and humane than just trying to alleviate the painful symptoms of disease. There is a huge difference between treating symptoms and health creation! Maybe you think there aren't any effective cures for your condition. I bet there are!

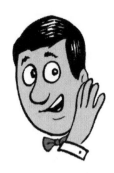

"Remember, health does not come from taking drugs. Health comes from proper nutrition and detoxification so that the body can heal itself. Unlike the 'pill for every ill' approach, creating an environment where the body can heal itself doesn't heal just one thing - it heals everything."

More and more studies are showing that heart disease, diabetes, hypertension, and cancer are diet and lifestyle related. If this is true, how can you cure them? Of course, change your diet and lifestyle!

1.5.1 The Check Engine Light

Let's say that the "check engine" light in your car came on and you took it to a mechanic to have it fixed. If he simply unplugged the light and said, "OK, no more check engine light." would he have fixed the problem? Of course not. The check engine light is just an indicator that something is wrong.

The same can be said for our health. Instead of just trying to control the symptoms, we need to address the underlying problem. If you get your blood glucose number under control, have you cured yourself of diabetes? No, an elevated blood sugar number is just a number. It's a symptom of the underlying disease. A healthy diet and moderate exercise will make you less insulin resistant.

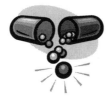

Certainly there is a place for pharmaceutical drugs in treating pain and the symptoms of some illnesses. I recently developed an infection in the cuticle of one of my fingers. I was hoping that my immune system would simply eliminate it, but it didn't. So I got a prescription for some antibiotics and, as shown in Figure 1-7, they knocked out the infection in just a few days. BUT it was the cells of my body that returned the finger back to normal. How can your body have the intelligence to automatically repair itself? I have no idea, but it does.

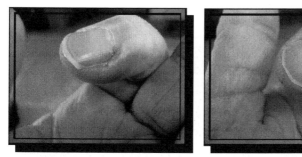

Figure 1-7 Before and After Finger Infection

On the other hand, I have been taking several different blood pressure medications. Eventually I became allergic to all of them! It's pretty scary when your tongue and throat swell up so you can't swallow and you think it might cut off your breathing. At the emergency room they just let it run its course, but they kept me there all day just incase they had to stick a tube down my throat. Not fun! Here are a few of the side effects listed right on the sheets that come with my blood pressure meds:

1. Serious (possibly fatal) liver problems
2. Confusion, mood swings or depression
3. Fainting
4. Irregular heartbeat
5. Yellowing eyes/skin
6. Persistent vomiting
7. Swelling of face, tongue or throat (This one I did experience)
8. Trouble breathing

If you listen to the ads on TV you will hear them list side effects for some medications that include:

1. Seizures
2. Liver, kidney, and lung damage
3. Skin irritation
4. Increased risk of serious infections
5. Increased risk of blood clots, heart attack, and stroke
6. Nerve damage and neuropathy
7. Cancer
8. Death

But they are quick to add, "Check with your doctor to see if this is right for you." I'm wondering how death can be right for you?

The large pharmaceutical companies aren't passionate about curing people; they are passionate about making money. They are in the business of treating symptoms, not finding and curing the cause. The simple fact is that there is no money in dead people, and there is no money in healthy people. The money is in people who are alive (sort of) but have chronic illnesses that require them to take medications for the rest of their lives.

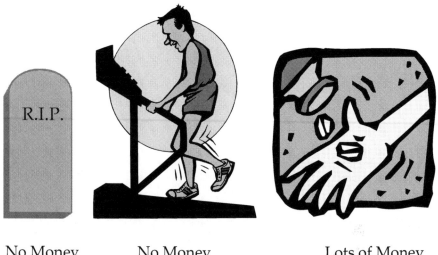

No Money   No Money   Lots of Money

Of course, any business should be allowed to make money, but many drugs are exorbitant. Also, the 5-year survival rate for stage 4 cancer patients receiving conventional treatment is only 2.1%. Only two out of a hundred survive for five years. Chemotherapy, surgery, and radiation aren't working! In fact, it is estimated that by 2020 over 50% of all cancer in America will be medically induced by drugs and radiation. We will look back in 20 or 30 years and be amazed that we actually used such barbaric treatments! There has to be a better way.

X-rays cause cancer, and CT scans are massive doses of radiation. Chemotherapy destroys the immune system, which is your only defense against cancer. Today in America we spend more on pharmaceuticals than ever before and we are sicker than ever before. This approach just isn't working.

So, what's the takeaway? Try to get well and eliminate as many medications as possible. I'm not saying to quit all of your medications right now. That would be foolish and dangerous. I am saying to try the nutritional approach and then, when you are well, through those meds in the trash can!

More and more studies have demonstrated that a plant-based, whole-foods diet will allow you to reduce or eliminate your prescription drugs.

Associated Press (May 14, 2008)
"Half of all insured Americans are taking prescription medicines regularly for chronic health problems."

1.5.3 The Nutritional Approach

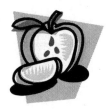

"Let your food be your medicine."
Hippocrates

What are the side effects of a plant-based diet?

1. Weight loss
2. Lower blood pressure
3. Lower cholesterol
4. More energy

5. Better health
6. Freedom

Why do I have "freedom" as a side effect of a plant-based diet? You are free of restrictions. The plant-based approach is simple. There is no calorie counting, and you can eat as much as you want. You are free from hunger, which is the thing that causes most people to quit their low-carb diets. Willpower only lasts so long. If you are in constant pain and crave calories, you will eventually quit the diet.

The standard American diet is calorie dense and nutrient deficient, but a high fiber, plant-based diet is nutrient dense and not deficient of anything.

1.5.4 The Incredible Human Body!

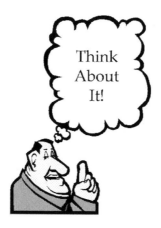

Think about it. When you get a cut, your body immediately starts to heal itself. You don't have to tell the individual cells what to do. In fact, if you could you wouldn't know what to tell them. How incredible is that! There is intelligence at the cellular level! All we have to do is create an environment that allows the body to heal itself.

It's not medications or nutrients that heal; they just help create an environment where the body can heal itself.

We live in a dirty world. We are constantly exposed to pathogens like viruses, bacteria and parasites. Your immune system is constantly fighting to keep you healthy. It's like two armies fighting a battle. Which one will win? If one side is strong and has superior weapons, they will win. Conversely, if the other side is weak, undernourished and has no weapons, they will loose. That's why doing all you can to boost your immune system is important. If you create an environment that makes it difficult for your body to heal itself you are in big trouble!

Now, I didn't cut myself on purpose so I could document it, but I happened to get a cut on my finger, so I figured I would take advantage of it to prove a point. Figure 1-8 shows the amazing healing that took place completely automatically.

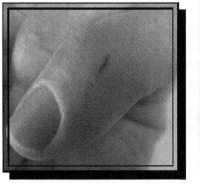
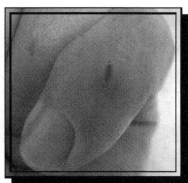

After One Day   After Three Days

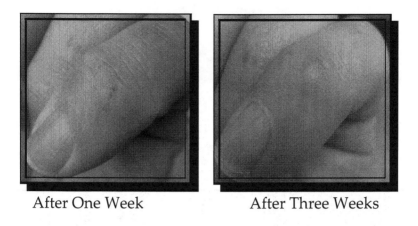

After One Week   After Three Weeks

Figure 1-8 Cut Healing Itself Automatically

Not to get too gross, but Figure 1-9 shows my tooth socket healing after an extraction. This was more serious than just a simple cut on the finger. The roots were so deep that they had grown right up into the sinus cavity. Without any antibiotics, my body was able to heal the wound. What an amazing and complex process! Again, the thing that amazes me the most is that this process took place completely automatically. If I had to consciously direct the healing process I wouldn't even know where to start!

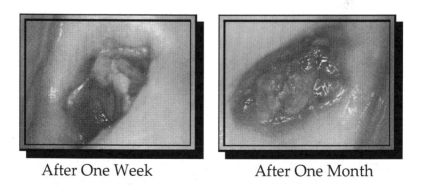

After One Week   After One Month

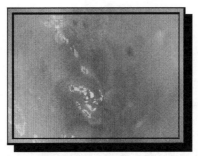

After Three Months

Figure 1-7 Tooth Socket Healing Itself

How amazing is that! A very complex healing process that my body performed automatically!

What can we do to make our immune system and our body's healing powers as strong as possible?

1. Don't smoke.
2. Eat a diet high in fruits and vegetables, not just to consume lots of nutrients for your cells, but also to nourish the "healthy bacteria" in your gut.
3. Get plenty of exercise, fresh air, and sunshine.
4. Maintain a healthy weight.
5. Keep a positive, optimistic attitude as much as possible. Expect good things to happen. Believe it or not, your emotions do affect your health.
6. Drink alcohol in moderation or not at all.
7. Give yourself permission to get plenty of sleep.
8. Avoid the toxins and dangerous chemicals that you find in packaged foods, household cleaning supplies, body wash and shampoo. There are safer alternatives. Read the ingredients labels on everything.
9. Take steps to avoid infection, such as washing your hands and face frequently. This is especially important if

you have the habit of rubbing your eyes (like I do). Think about it. If someone sneezes into their hands and then wants to shake your hand, they may as well have sneezed directly in your face. Do you know what's on the handle of your shopping cart? You may be surprised! I always wipe the handle down when antibiotic wipes are available, and I wash my hands and face as soon as I get home.

10. Avoid using antibiotics as much as possible. They also kill off the good bacteria. Of course, there are times when the proper use of antibiotics can save your life, but let your immune system take care of most colds and minor infections.

11. Minimize stress.

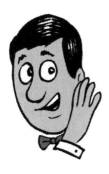

"You'll notice that the things that strengthen your immune system are also the things help that cure any disease."

1.6 Get Educated and Have a Plan

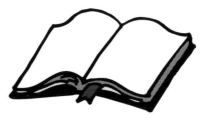

How can you get educated about foods, drugs, and lifestyle options? There is a wealth of information available. The only problem is that much of it is conflicting. Who can you believe?

1.6.1 Who Can You Believe?

Here are a few questions to ask:

1. Are there valid, peer-reviewed studies supporting the claim?
2. Is the study or video documentary real? Are there real people (not just actors) involved?
3. Who paid for the study? Are there conflicts of interest involved? Did the National Pharmaceutical Council, the Beef Board, or the Egg Board sponsor the study? If so, you can bet they have influenced the results.
4. Was the "expert scientist" who approved the study compensated? If so, by whom?
5. Are lobbyists involved?

Finding reliable information may seem like an uphill battle because of the profit motive. Big pharma, industrial farming, and food manufacturing companies understand that there are huge profits to be made. They will protect their interests by any means available to them.

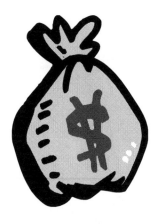

Now, I may be overly optimistic, but I think I see a popular movement growing that supports holistic medicine and nutrition for wellness. Almost all of the documentaries on FMTV have actual MD's who have discovered things they never learned in medical school, and they are excited about promoting health instead of just treating symptoms with drugs.

I told my doctor at the VA about the nutritional approach I am taking, and instead of saying, "Nutrition has nothing to do with it" he told me about a friend of his who cured himself of diabetes with a Vegan diet. I think doctors are starting to become aware.

Let's face it; industrial food production and pharmaceuticals are big business. The average person doesn't realize how large and powerful these organizations are. Don't think their goal is to get you healthy. Their goal is to make as much money as possible.

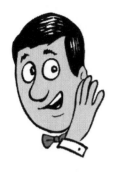 *"Health makes sense, but it doesn't make dollars."*

In Appendix A, I present a fairly extensive list of resources, but to get you started immediately let me just mention Food Matters TV (FMTV). There is a subscription fee, but I consider it a bargain. They have an extensive collection of documentary videos and a helpful Facebook group. You can consider them the "Netflix for Health." Visit fmtv.com and check them out.

Also, if you are already a Netflix subscriber, you will find several excellent documentaries there. Some of my favorites include **Forks Over Knives**, **The C Word**, **In Defense of Food**, and **What the Health**.

1.6.2 Take Charge of Your Own Health

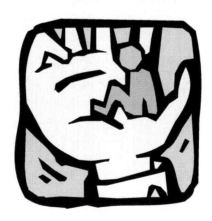

Somehow we have come to believe that you need to do what your doctor tells you. After all, he's the one with all the medical training. What do I know? You need to take responsibility for your own health. Don't just turn it over to him and blindly follow whatever advice you are given. There are many brilliant and concerned health care professionals out there, but you need to play an active role in your health care.

It's not that you will disagree with your doctor (you might at times), but your success will be much greater if you take responsibility for your health, and are an **active participant** in your healing. You can't just give someone else some money and say, "You fix me."

Today there is a huge amount of information available for free on the Internet regarding health and nutrition. Can reading articles, watching videos, or attending health and wellness retreat workshops make you more knowledgeable that your doctor? Of course, not, but "The times they are a' changing."

We're in a transitional period (2019 at this writing). Medical schools are slow to change their curriculum from "drugs for treating symptoms" to "nutrition and lifestyle changes for promoting health." They need to add in many more courses that explain how diet and lifestyle changes affect health.

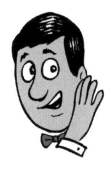

"Promoting health and preventing chronic diseases will enhance the lives of millions of people, and it will save our medical system from bankruptcy."

Today patients have a wealth of new information regarding health available to them. The challenge is to sort out the good information from commercial advertisements (which there are plenty!). The traditional medical school pharmaceutical approach is gradually giving way to a more holistic approach. This approach is based on preventing disease and curing those who have a chronic disease instead of just treating their symptoms for the rest of their (miserable) lives. You can see changes taking place even on the websites of the American Cancer Society https://www.cancer.org/ and the American Medical Association https://www.ama-assn.org/

1.6.3 Keep It Simple

The goal of everything I recommend in this book is to help you be successful in your quest for better health. Simple is good. You can always add more complexity to your program once it is working for you, but at first keep it simple. This means:

1. Set goals that you can write down in a few words, and that are easy to understand.
2. Keep your goals limited to just a few - not everything you can possibly imagine. If your goal list has three or four items, that's a good thing. If your goal list has 100 items, you will give up and quit!

1.6.4 Make It Real

Your goals need to be realistic and achievable. Otherwise you are guaranteed to fail. It's not your fault; nobody can achieve unrealistic goals. Either you will get frustrated and quit or you will keep trying the rest of your life and not reach that unachievable goal.

Start out with a meal plan and an exercise plan that you can actually do. It's good to push yourself a little as you make progress, but start out with an easy and enjoyable program.

1. If walking is your preferred exercise, start out with slow, short walks at first. Distance and speed will come naturally.
2. If you are doing some training with weights, start out with just a few exercises and add a few more as time goes on. Also, use light weights at first.
3. Choose meals that are enjoyable and easy to prepare.
4. Don't get caught up with unrealistic expectations.

Have you ever seen an advertisement with a superstar model demonstrating a piece of equipment or selling a certain product? The implication is, "If you join this gym or eat this thing, you will look like me." The ad might be enjoyable to watch, but it's:

Not gonna' happen!

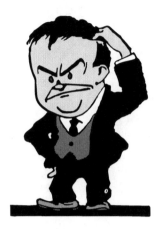

If you are starting on this healthy diet and lifestyle program, you are going to be making some major decisions. That's great! But keep the following in mind:

1.7.1 Quick Fix vs. Permanent Change

It's exciting to see rapid change in your health, and this plan will bring fairly rapid change, but this program is not a quick fix. So, don't be discouraged if progress is slow at first. This is a plan that you can live with for the rest of your life!

1.7.2 The Treadmill Fiasco

Shortly after my trip to the emergency room my doctor ordered a stress test. They got me all hooked up, but I only lasted a couple of minutes and didn't even get off the first level. Figure 1-8 shows my feeble attempt at the treadmill. How embarrassing!

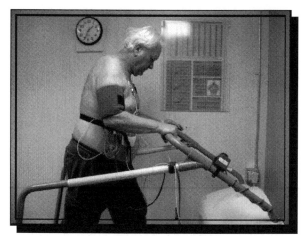

Figure 1-8 The Treadmill Fiasco

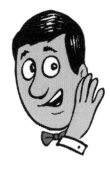

"If you keep doing what you have always done, You will keep getting what you always get."

1.7.3 Make a List

Just thinking about your goals can be exciting, but if you want to make them concrete, write them down. I'm not sure why it works, but it does.

Write down your goals. Be as **specific** as possible, and include a **timeframe** for achieving them. It's more important to have a list of goals than it is to actually achieve them! That may sound contradictory, but formalizing your goals is where it starts. If you fall short, you will achieve them eventually.

1.8 How to Lower Your Blood Pressure

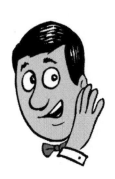

Important Note:
*"Eliminating all prescription medications is an excellent goal, but until you can get your hypertension down naturally, keep taking your blood pressure meds. The important thing is to make sure that your blood pressure is under control in the mean time. You don't want to have a stroke before you get it into the safe zone. A big stroke can do **permanent** damage. Consult with your doctor before dropping (or even reducing) your meds."*

High blood pressure is "non-symptomatic" because a person with high blood pressure doesn't feel anything unless he is having a stroke or it is high enough to cause a headache. That's why it is called the "silent killer."

1.8.1 My Water Hose Analogy

If a water hose has too much pressure it will burst. Same thing for the blood vessels in your brain! If you pinch off a hose, the water won't flow. The same thing happens with a blood clot in your arteries. High blood pressure can damage your liver and your kidneys. If you've ever seen someone who has had a stroke, you know that's something you don't want! Are you with me on this? We're talking serious stuff here!

These blood pressure lowering tips may seem obvious, but I never thought about them until I was in trouble myself. Things can get out of control; I mean actually out of your control. That's a bad situation believe me.

These are tips that everyone should follow even though they don't have hypertension.

1. Increase the amount of plant-based foods you are consuming. Include as many dark, rich colors (phytochemicals) as possible, and cut out junk food.
2. Reduce your salt intake.
3. Achieve and then maintain a healthy weight.
4. Exercise regularly.
5. Limit alcohol.
6. Quit smoking.
7. Drink plenty of water.
8. Find a way to manage stress.
9. Take time for some slow deep breathing each day.

1.9 Here's My Plan

Based on what I have learned about nutrition and lifestyle, I have devised a plan that I can follow for the rest of my lift. It may change somewhat as time goes on, but here's my plan for right now. Your plan may be a little different. You may not include some of the things that I feel are important, and you may add in some things that I'm missing. That's perfectly fine! We each need a plan that we can live with for a lifetime.

So, here are the pillars of my health program.

1.9.1 Sobriety

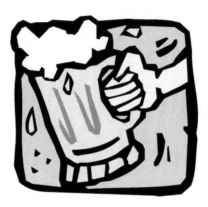

I have drunk beer all of my adult life. In the past several years since I have been living alone, my beer consumption has been a 12-pack almost every day. I really enjoy it, but you know that can't be good for your health.

The beer had to go!

It's not that I got into trouble or drove my car while drinking. I just drank by myself at home while working on the computer or watching TV. But that much alcohol had to be damaging my liver and kidneys. Also, it boosted my blood pressure sky high. A 12-pack of my favorite beer has 1716 calories (that's 143 calories per 12 oz can), and when I was drinking I wasn't concerned about healthy living. Of course, I didn't take my blood pressure meds. Sad but true!

You wouldn't believe the crazy things my alcoholic thinking led me to do. I used to double bag my trash or put it in a black trash bag just so the neighbors wouldn't see how many beer cans I was throwing out.

Does digging through the trash to retrieve the beers that I threw out earlier that morning sound like rational behavior?

I have tried to quit drinking **hundreds** of times without success. Finally I'm at the point where I have no choice. This program is A COMPLETE LIFE CHANGE. That's one of my keys to success.

When I was young I used to smoke cigarettes. I was completely addicted, and I loved to have a pack of cigarettes rolled up in the sleeve of my T-shirt (OK, you probably have to be old to understand that). I smoked two packs a day and was completely powerless to quit. It took a major life change for me to get off the smokes. I thank God for His intervention way back then. Fast-forward 50 years, and here I am today dealing with food and alcohol addictions! I'm 75 years old, but would like to live a few more years in relatively good health and share some of my passions with others. Then, when it comes time to wrap things up, I'll be at peace.

Like smoking or food addiction, alcohol addiction isn't just one habit. It's linked to almost every activity in my life. That's why this program is not just about diet and exercise - it is a complete life change!

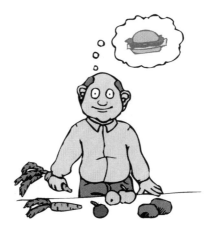

As I have said elsewhere, you don't have to adopt a vegetarian or Vegan lifestyle to benefit from this program. That's just my personal choice. Going Vegan "all the way" to me seems like the simplest way. I think for me it takes a complete life change to be effective for the long term.

Adopting a whole-foods, plant-based diet will help you regain your health.

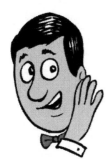

Regarding a plant-based diet, Dr. Alan Goldhamer, founder of TrueNorth Health Center (which has helped over 10,000 people regain their health) says, "It never doesn't work."

If becoming vegetarian seems too extreme, just start introducing more fruits and vegetables into your diet. Eventually the good stuff will push out the bad stuff.

1.9.3 Avoid Toxins as Much as Possible

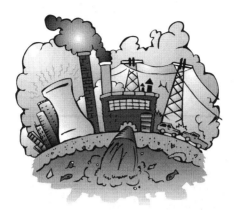

We are continually exposed to toxins in the air, the water, and in our food. We don't even think about it, but our immune system is constantly waging war against toxins and other "invaders" that don't belong in our bodies. Think about the army of workers that is protecting you from bacteria, viruses, parasites, cancer cells, and harmful chemical compounds. They work all the time, 24 hours a day to keep you safe. Wow! You have someone on your side! Doesn't it make sense to give them all the tools they need and not overload them with work they don't need to do?

Many toxins we can't avoid, but some we can. We can determine what foods we eat and what type of household products we use. We have complete control over what we purchase with our hard-earned dollars. And, by the way, it's you and me who govern the market by the way we spend our money.

What about the water we drink? Our bodies are about two thirds water, so this is an important topic. We can exclude lots of things from our diet, but we can't live very long without water. Our local governments are looking out for our health by putting fluorine and chlorine into our drinking water. The concept of killing off pathogens in our drinking water is a good one, but once this treated water reaches our homes we need to filter out these harmful chemicals. The "last mile" is up to us as individuals.

For many years I have used a simple carbon filter to make tap water taste better, but Figure 1-9 shows the Home Master F2 countertop filter that I just purchased. Besides dirt and microbes, it will remove chemicals such as fluoride and chlorine. It wasn't expensive, but produces clean, health promoting water.

So, we get the best of both worlds. Let the city clean up the water and then we filter out the harmful chemicals with our own filtration system.

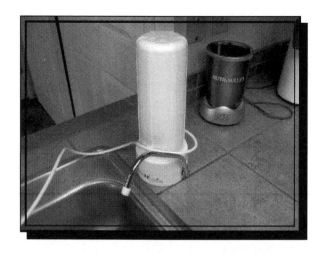

Figure 1-9 Home Master F2 Water Filter

A recent FDA report indicates that a chemical coating used in microwave popcorn bags breaks down when heated into a substance called perfluorooctanoic (PFOA). The Environmental Protection Agency has identified PFOA as a likely carcinogen. Another good reason to use an air popper or some healthy oil on the stovetop.

It's obvious that what you eat and drink is going to end up in your body, but much of what you put on your skin will end up in your body too. Your skin is not an impenetrable barrier. So, think about your shampoo, body wash, household cleaning supplies, etc. If you have to wear rubber gloves to use a cleaning product, you know it can't be good for you! Most toxins won't kill you right away, but they can build up in your system (bioaccumulation) and can impair your immune function.

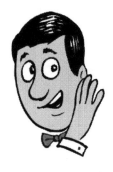

"Your immune system is your friend. Treat him well."

I always buy laundry detergent, body wash, and hand lotion that say "Fragrance Free - Hypoallergenic." That may not be enough, but it's a start. Legally manufacturers don't have to tell us what's in their fragrances, and many times these fragrances have lots of chemicals - many of them toxic.

Ladies put cosmetics directly on their lips and faces. Men (sometimes) use deodorants on their underarms. Years ago as a young engineer I did a network installation at one of the Dial Corp. facilities. The guy I was working with casually mentioned that there is a difference between a deodorant and an antiperspirant. An antiperspirant is considered to be a drug because it reacts with the body. So it falls under different rules. I thought that was amazing. I had never considered it before.

What is the main ingredient in most antiperspirants, and many antacids? Aluminum. When we think about heavy metal poising we usually think about lead, but aluminum in your system is heavy metal poisoning! So, think about your deodorant. Is that nitpicking? Heavy metal poising creates brain damage. Figure 1-10 is a picture of the backside of my (used to be) favorite toothpaste. Check out the warning.

> If more than used for brushing is accidentally swallowed, get medical help or contact a **POISON CONTROL CENTER** right away.

OK, this warning is meant primarily for children, but if it is poison for children, can it be good for us?

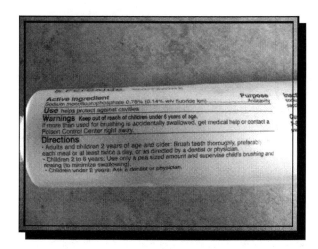

Figure 1-10 My (used to be) Favorite Toothpaste

Today there is a big debate regarding GMOs (Genetically Modified Organisms). Europe is much more strict than America in prohibiting the use of GMOs. The question about the health effects of GMOs is not yet settled, and probably won't be for several years to come. If you take a gene from one species and splice it into a different species can you guarantee the long-term health effect on people who eat that food? Can you guarantee what future generations of that GMO species are going to look like?

79

This is scary stuff, and that's why I put the whole topic of GMOs in this toxins section. For right now I consider GMOs as toxic substances. I know that eliminates lots of currently available products, but I'd rather just eliminate them than take chances with my health. There are plenty of non-GMO options still available today (that could change as large agribusiness takes over the entire food system).

1.9.4 Exercise

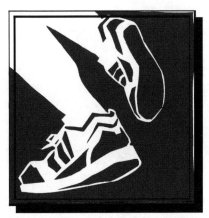

Get Moving!

Exercise is wonderful for improving your physical and emotional health! It stimulates your cardiovascular system, your muscles, your joints and ligaments. It massages your feet and increases blood flow. Just taking a walk does all these things!

You can't exercise off a bad diet, so don't even think about exercise as a weight loss tool. Don't think about how many miles you have to run to burn off a specific number of calories. That approach is a loosing battle. You would have to do an extreme amount of exercise to burn off any significant amount of calories. Just forget about that and let your metabolism take care of burning the calories. Your body will naturally bring your weight down to the ideal level.

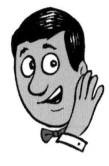

"Think about exercise as a wonderful healthy activity in its own right. Do it because it is good for you!"

When I was at my highest weight I didn't exercise at all because it was painful just to walk. I would struggle just to get from the bedroom to the living room! I would grab hold of everything along the way for support and just to keep my balance. After loosing only ten pounds I was able to walk much better.

Everybody is different regarding the type of exercise they prefer. Choose something you enjoy. If you don't enjoy it, you won't keep it up very long. I like hiking. I enjoy the peace and quiet of the beautiful hiking trails in the Bradshaw Mountains of Prescott, Arizona. So, hiking is my exercise of choice. It is low-impact, enjoyable, and meditative.

I have a set of dumbbells for upper body toning. I'm sure there will come a point when I'll start using them. Again, to make it interesting I will keep track of the weights and "reps" for each exercise.

1.9.5 Watch Health Videos and Inspirational Stories

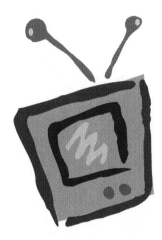

I watch a health video or inspiring story every day for education and motivation. There are several good ones on Netflix, and a large collection on FMTV. My favorite ones are documentaries about real people (average people like you and me) making changes in their lives. I list several of my favorites in Appendix A.

1.9.6 Keep a Diary or Write a Book

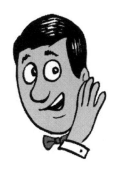

"Just working on this book each day is very motivating for me."

You may think, "I'm not a writer." but writing a book, keeping a journal, or starting a blog is a great way to document your journey. Also, it is an excellent way to commit to this program. It is a way to become accountable to yourself and to others. I bet you will enjoy reading through your journal years from now (even the parts where you slipped or took a few steps backward). If you start a website or a blog, you can share your journey with thousands of other people!

You may write something that is helpful or inspiring to others. Getting spontaneous feedback from people saying how you helped them is such a wonderful experience!

1.9.7 Plan for a Major Event

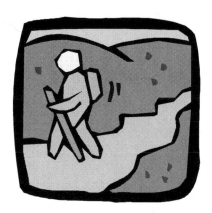

If you are working towards a major goal it will inspire you to keep after your health program. Choose a goal that is a challenge, but not too far out of reach. You want to actually be able to accomplish it in a reasonable length of time. You can always set more ambitious goals later, but for now pick one that you know you will be able to accomplish. Maybe you want to run a 10K race, improve your golf score, or climb a mountain.

1.9.8 Relaxation and Visualization

Which of the following images portrays your current situation?

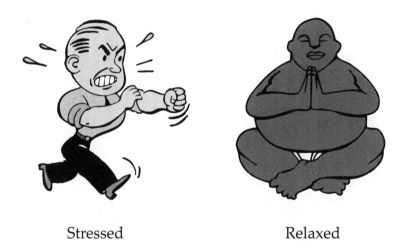

Stressed   Relaxed

Relaxation, meditation, visualization, and prayer may seem like mysterious subjects, but like everything else I do, I try to keep it pretty simple. I just sit in my comfortable recliner, relax, and picture myself as I want to be. Visualization is a way to program your subconscious mind. I have an old photograph of myself when I was young and in great shape. So I visualize looking like that. You might ask, "You think you can get back into the shape you were when you were young?" Well, why not? I can certainly look and feel a lot more like that than I do today!

84

I have a technique for relaxation that you might like. Once I am settled into my recliner I do the following:

1. I consciously relax each part of my body my saying, "Relax your face; now relax your neck and shoulders; relax your arms and hands; etc" until I have relaxed every part of my body.

2. Then I say, "Now you are completely relaxed. You are gently drifting down like a leaf in the forest. Just drifting down . . ."

3. At that point I am very relaxed and ready to picture myself as thin and strong. I also visualize all of my organs functioning at peak performance and my blood pressure monitor showing a nice low reading in the normal range.

The whole process doesn't take more than 10 - 15 minutes. Don't rush it. Just enjoy the experience of feeding these images to your subconscious. When you are finished, you will feel refreshed and ready to get on with your life.

Athletes use visualization all the time to increase their performance. You may not be planning on going to the Olympics, but you can use visualization to achieve your goals.

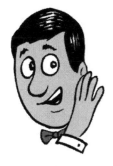

"What you think about you bring about."

We are learning more every day about the mind/body connection. Emotions are more than just electrical activity in the brain. Various emotions cause the release of chemicals into the blood stream. Some of these chemicals are damaging to healthy cells, and some are beneficial. Adrenaline helps us through dangerous situations in the short term, but chronic stress and the continuous release of adrenaline is harmful.

Negative emotions and stress cause a release of cortisol, which inhibits the immune system, making us more vulnerable to disease. Positive emotions suppress the release of this stress hormone and promote health. This is a huge topic that we are just starting to understand, but the bottom line is that there is a very real, chemical connection between emotions and the body.

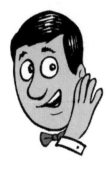

"Pessimists may be right more often, but optimist live longer."

No wonder we have sayings like "Laughter is good medicine."

1.9.9 Record Your Stats Every Day

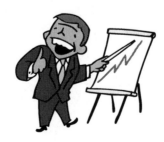

Keeping track of my blood pressure and weight on a daily basis is motivating to me. Table 1-1 below makes it easy for me to record these stats every day.

Month:					
Date	BP	Weight	Date	BP	Weight
1			17		
2			18		
3			19		
4			20		
5			21		
6			22		
7			23		
8			24		
9			25		
10			26		
11			27		
12			28		
13			29		
14			30		
15			31		
16					

Table 1-1 Blood Pressure Log

Chapter 2. The Lowdown on Foods

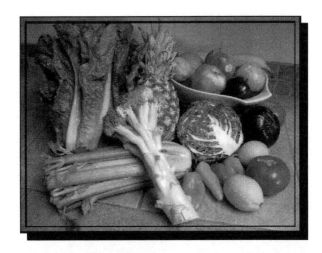

2.1 The Standard American Diet

Today in America we are suffering an epidemic of obesity, heart disease, diabetes and cancer because people are eating the Standard American Diet (SAD) that is loaded with fat, salt, sugar and chemicals. Instead of eating a diet high in fruits, vegetables, nuts, seeds, whole grains and beans we are eating a diet of "food like" products that are processed and prepackaged. These products and loaded with chemicals, toxins, antibiotics and pesticides. The goal of our industrial food system is not to produce healthy food but to produce profits. It is so pervasive that even in hospital waiting rooms the vending machines have candy bars and potato chips. You would think that hospitals would be places that promote health!

A recent phenomenon is the rapid rise in childhood obesity and diabetes. If children contract these diseases early, they will be very sick as adults!

Right now (2019) half of the American population has diabetes or are pre-diabetic, and this epidemic will only get worse without a popular revolution in the way we think about food.

Our ancient ancestors lived at a time when food was scarce and hard to get. They were driven by their brain chemistry to eat as much cholerically dense food as they could so they would survive long enough to reproduce. We are still wired that way today. Our DNA hasn't changed that much from theirs, but the available food supply has! Today there is an abundance of processed foods containing loads of the fat, sugar, and salt that we have been programmed to crave.

The key for us today is to eat real food. Eat plants, not food that was manufactured in a plant. If you buy food that comes in a box you would be better off to throw the contents out and eat the box! OK, maybe I'm being a little bit melodramatic, but the idea is to eat unprocessed foods that come from nature, not from a factory.

Many traditional cultures that eat a primarily plant-based diet have virtually no cancer or heart disease. Once they start eating the American diet they rapidly get as overweight and sick as we are. Their DNA didn't change; their diet and lifestyle are the things that changed. That's pretty good evidence that we are not completely controlled by our genetics. So, don't feel you are a helpless victim of your genetic makeup and there is nothing you can do about it. Even if you have a genetic predisposition toward certain diseases, if those genes are not "turned on" by an unhealthy environment in your body, you may never get the disease. Today we are starting to understand a lot more about "epigenetics" and how genes are expressed.

Genetics is like playing poker; you may have been dealt a good hand or a bad hand. You can't change your genome, but you can change how it is expressed. So forget about genetics and just play the hand you were dealt.

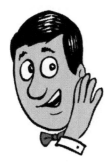

"Another thing to consider is that we don't just pass down our genetics, we also pass down our habits to our kids."

2.1.1 The Pleasure Trap

Hunger and cravings are not the same thing. As an alcoholic I have cravings to drink beer because it stimulates the pleasure centers in my brain. I'm not a neuroscientist so I don't know exactly how it happens, but the alcohol somehow interferes with the neurotransmitters in my brain. Drinking alcohol has no real benefits except for creating an amazing feeling of pleasure. It somehow triggers the release of dopamine in my brain. For me its drawbacks far outweigh that temporary sense of well-being.

The same thing can be said for eating junk food that is loaded with sugar, salt and fat. It has the same effect in our brains as alcohol or other drugs. If we still lived in a time of feast or famine, eating as much high-choleric food as we could might work to our advantage. We would store the extra calories as fat to get us through the lean times, but today for most of us, there are no lean times so we just keep storing the extra calories as fat. Plus, modern packaged foods contain chemical toxins, preservatives, dies and carcinogens.

So what's the difference between cravings and hunger? Real hunger is a good thing. It encourages us to consume nutrients that promote health, but cravings are a desire to eat and drink stuff so we can temporarily feel good. Then we are using food as entertainment.

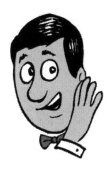

"We need to view eating as consuming the healthy nutrients that our bodies need, not as entertainment. We can still take pleasure in eating, but we will also have the satisfaction of knowing that what we are eating is good for us."

2.1.2 Fats

Fats have gotten a bad rap, but fats are essential for health. They are part of the myelin sheath that surrounds nerve cells and allows them to send electrical signals. Our brains contain large amounts of fat. In fact, fat is an essential component in the cell membranes of all of our cells. It is also an essential part of hormones that regulate many bodily functions.

We store the extra calories that we don't burn right away in fat cells (adipose tissue) so that it will be available during the lean times. The problem today is that we keep storing fat, but we don't have any lean times to burn it off!

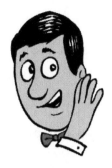

"You've probably heard about low-fat/high-carb diets
And high-fat/low-carb diets. How confusing!
How about a balanced diet with the right amount of
fat and carbs?
It's called a whole-foods, plant-based diet."

2.2 Plant-based Nutrition

Plant-based nutrition is "clean" with no animal growth hormones, excessive fat, cholesterol or antibiotics. Eating a wide variety of colorful plants gives you all the nutrients you need except for vitamin D and B-12. The multi vitamin that I take has plenty of each.

The FDA has proposed several different food pyramids over the years. Figure 2-1 is my proposal. Notice that there is no room for processed foods or animal products. Let's start eating a healthy, clean and compassionate diet!

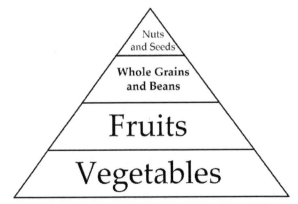

Figure 2-1 Rick McKeon's Healthy Food Pyramid

2.2.1 What About Protein?

One of the most common questions people ask about a vegetarian diet is, "Where do you get your protein and calcium?"

The meat and dairy industries have spent a lot of money trying to convince the American public that meat and dairy products are necessary in order to ensure that we have enough protein and calcium for good health. But the reality is that if you eat a variety of fruits, vegetables, nuts, seeds, whole grains and beans there's no way you will be deficient in any of the essential nutrients. The key is to eat a VARIETY of COLORFUL fruits and vegetables.

Good sources of plant protein include: Lentils, black beans, lima beans, peanuts, wild rice, chickpeas, almonds, chia seeds, oatmeal, cashews, pumpkin seeds, potatoes, spinach, organic corn, avocado, broccoli, Brussels sprouts, spirulina, green peas, hemp seeds, zucchini, collard greens, kale, flaxseeds, organic edamame, sunflower seeds, and walnuts.

2.2.2 What About Calcium?

Good sources of dietary calcium include: Kale, mustard greens, collard greens, broccoli, black beans, chia seeds, sesame seeds, almonds, fennel, oranges, blackberries and figs.

2.2.3 What About Vitamins B-12 and D?

Of the thirteen essential vitamins, plants don't provide vitamins B-12 or D-3. For those I supplement with a multivitamin. There are plenty of high quality inexpensive multivitamins available. The one shown in Figure 2-2 has 1,667% of the minimum daily requirement for B-12 and 500% of vitamin D-3.

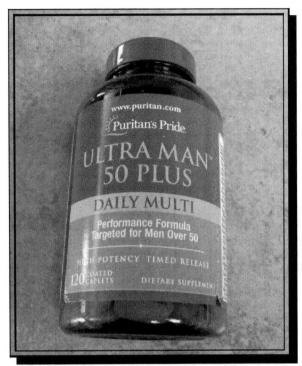

Figure 2-2 Typical Multivitamin

2.3 Animal Based Nutrition

As I stated earlier, I am not asking you to give up meat and dairy entirely, but when considering animal based nutrition consider the following.

2.3.1 Things to Consider

1. The International Agency for Research on Cancer (IARC), which is the cancer agency of the World Health Organization, classifies processed meat as a Group 1

carcinogen. Processed meat includes hot dogs, ham, bacon, sausage, and some deli meats.

2. Many processed meats are pink in color because they are injected with sodium nitrite - a known carcinogen.
3. All animal products contain high levels of fat, cholesterol, and growth hormones.
4. Animal flesh has no fiber, and in many cases contains antibiotics and puss.
5. Meat, eggs, and dairy products are high in cholesterol and saturated fat.
6. Eating meat can increase your risk for cancer, osteoporosis, and heart disease.
7. Eating meat will drive up your insulin levels.
8. Industrial feedlots are so unsanitary that the cows are fed antibiotics. This makes a perfect breeding ground for super strains of bacteria.
9. If you ever get a glimpse inside industrial animal production you would be appalled!

2.3.2 Cow's Milk

Cow's milk is the perfect food . . . for baby cows. Even calves stop drinking cow's milk at a certain point and start eating grass. In the same way, human babies stop drinking mothers' milk at a certain point, and don't need to switch over to cow's milk. They don't need any milk after weaning.

Drinking cow's milk sets up an acidic condition in the blood. To neutralize this acidity your body draws calcium from your bones. Contrary to the marketing hype that you need to drink milk for strong bones; those populations who drink the most milk have the highest incidence of osteoporosis.

Industrial animal production is not only horrific in terms of cruelty, but it produces more greenhouse gasses and pollution than the entire transportation sector.

"Let the good stuff push out the bad stuff."

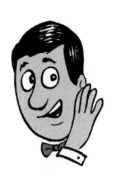

"My approach is to jump in with both feet, but if you are new to the plant-based approach and are still craving junk food, just try adding in more fruits and vegetables. The more healthy food you consume, the less junk food you will crave. Maybe for you it will be a gradual process."

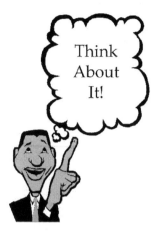

Whole foods are foods that are "whole." That may seem obvious, but think about it. Foods that are highly processed and come in a package are not whole foods. If you read the ingredients label on the package you will notice lots of added sugar, preservatives, and some chemicals that you can't even pronounce. Stay away from prepackaged, processed foods!

Of course processed foods taste great. Why, because they have been engineered to taste great. That usually involves adding salt, sugar, and fat.

2.4.1 Food Should Be Grown, Not Manufactured

Most manufactured foods aren't really "food" - they are "food like substances." There may be pictures of food on the box, but that's not what's in the box. Maybe the ingredients started out as real food, but they have been processed to death and have all kinds of chemicals added.

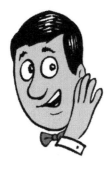

"There's no such thing as 'junk food.' There's food and there's junk."

Not all foods that come in a bag or a can are bad for you. What we're looking for is minimal processing with no added chemicals, salt, or sugar. In other words, foods that are as close to nature as possible.

Figures 2-3 through 2-6 show some prepackaged foods that are healthy. Frozen foods are generally regarded as just as healthy as fresh. The nutrients are still there and no preservatives have been added. Notice that each of these has only one ingredient - the vegetable itself.

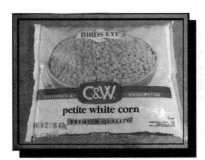 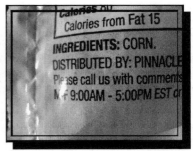

Figure 2-3 Frozen Corn

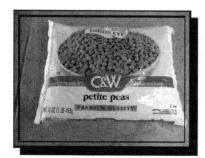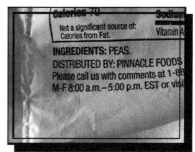

Figure 2-4 Frozen Peas

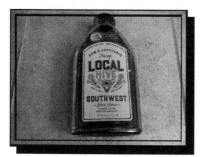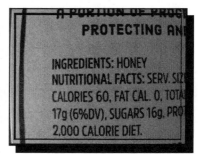

Figure 2-5 Raw Honey

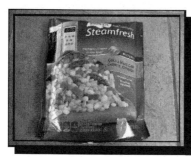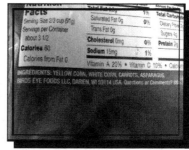

Figure 2-6 Birds Eye Steamfresh Vegetable Mixture

If you pick up a banana or a zucchini squash in the grocery store you won't see an ingredients label. It is what it is. Try to eat foods the way they came up out of the ground.

Be leery of anything that has an ingredients panel, especially if it takes up the whole side of the box or has words on it that you can't pronounce. Which is easier to pronounce, "apple" or "disodium inosinate"?

By the way, the Microsoft Word spell checker recognized "apple" but flagged "disodium inosinate" as a spelling error.

Below are the ingredients panels from three products. Figure 2-7 is from a jar of organic almond butter. Figure 2-8 is from a box of Old-Fashioned oats, and Figure 2-9 is from a box of veggie hot dogs. See the difference?

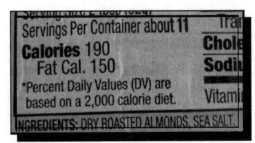

Figure 2-7 Organic Almond Butter (Two Ingredients)

INGREDIENTS: 100% ROLLED OATS.
DISTRIBUTED BY
BETTER LIVING BRANDS LLC
P.O. BOX 99
PLEASANTON, CA 94566-0009
1-888-723-3929
www.betterlivingbrandsLLC.com

Figure 2-8 Old-Fashioned Oats (One Ingredient)

Ingredients: Water, wheat gluten, corn syrup solids, contains two percent or less of methylcellulose, dextrose, salt, egg whites, natural flavors, brown sugar (sugar, molasses), hydrolyzed vegetable protein (corn protein, soy protein), hydrolyzed corn protein, soy protein isolate, carrageenan, mustard flour, onion powder, maltodextrin, spices, xanthan gum, hydrolyzed soy protein, autolyzed yeast, paprika, garlic powder, soybeans, disodium guanylate, disodium inosinate, hydrolyzed torula and brewers yeast, wheat, gum arabic, hydrolyzed vegetable protein (corn gluten, soy protein, wheat gluten), soybean oil, thiamin hydrochloride, paprika extract for color, autolyzed yeast extract, lactic acid, nonfat milk, red 40, sunflower oil, citric acid, blue 1.
CONTAINS WHEAT, EGG, SOY AND MILK INGREDIENTS.

Figure 2-9 Veggie Hot Dogs (Vegan Junk Food)

There is such a thing as Vegan junk food! It may not contain animal products (actually these veggie dogs do), but they are processed foods with added chemicals.

2.4.3 Don't Let the Picture Fool You!

When I saw the label of Figure 4-10 on a jar of mayonnaise I thought, "This should be healthy. It is made from avocado." But if you read the ingredients label you will discover that it has some avocado oil in it, but that is just one of many ingredients including other oils, chemical preservatives, and eggs.

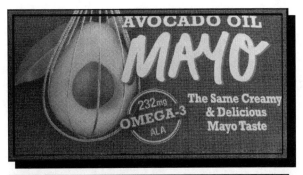

Figure 2-10 "Avocado" Mayonnaise

This is just for fun, but it makes a point about some of the stuff we consume. Most people wouldn't recognize many of these words. So, are we describing foods or a mixture of chemicals? Can you guess what these products are based on their ingredients? Some will be easier than others. You will find the answers in Appendix B.

1. butylparaben, hypromellose, microcrystalline cellulose and carboxymethylcellulose sodium, potassium citrate, propylparaben, simethicone emulsion, sorbitol, aluminum hydroxide, magnesium hydroxide.

2. salt, sugar, monosodium glutamate, maltodextrin, hydrolyzed corn, wheat and soy protein, turmeric, lactose, dehydrated vegetables, disodium inosinate, disodium guanylate, vegetable oil, yeast extract, powdered cooked chicken, reduced iron, TBHQ, potassium carbonate, sodium (mono, hexameta, and/or tripoly) phosphate, sodium carbonate.

3. textured vegetable protein, corn oil, sunflower oil, egg whites, corn starch, soy protein isolate, autolyzed yeast extract, salt, caramel color, onion powder, hydrolyzed vegetable protein, garlic powder, potato starch, maltodextrin, disodium guanylate, disodium inosinate, succinic acid, sugar, nonfat dry milk, soybean oil, wheat fiber.

4. apple

5. enriched wheat flower, thiamine mononitrate, soybean oil, salt, sugar, yeast, corn syrup, palm oil, cornmeal, wheat semolina, datem, wheat gluten, dextrose, guar gum, calcium pyrophosphate, hydrogenated soybean oil,

wheat protein isolate, sodium bicarbonate, sodium aluminum phosphate, olive oil, l-cysteine, annatto, xanthan gum.

6. water, glycerin, cocamidopropyl betaine, sodium laureth sulfate, sodium hydrolyzed potato starch, dodecenylsuccinate, Avena sativa kernel flour, citric acid, sodium benzoate, guar hydroxypropyltimonium chloride, tetrasodium glutamate diacetate, dipropylene glycol, glycol distearate, polyquaternium-10, acrylates/C10-30 alkyl acrylate crosspolymer, laureth-4, PEG-20 almond glycerides, sodium hydroxide, coriandrum sativum fruiy oil, Avena sativa kernel oil, commiphora myrrha oil, elettaria cardamomum seed oil, Avena sativa kernel extract.

7. banana

8. Idaho potatoes, vegetable oil, corn syrup solids, salt, maltodextrin, nonfat dry milk, sugar, sodium caseinate, butter powder, annatto color, disodium phosphate, momo and diglycerides, calcium stearoyl lactylate, natural and artificial flavors, spice, sodium acid pyrophosphate, sodium bisulfite, mixed tocopherols, silicon dioxide.

9. organic popcorn kernels

2.5 Conventional vs. Organic: There Is a Difference!

A lot of people would like you to believe there is no difference between conventional and organically grown foods. After all, they are genetically the same plant except for genetically modified organisms (GMOs).

But the difference is in how they are grown. The two major differences involve what is sprayed on them and the type of soil they are grown in.

2.5.1 Pesticides, Herbicides, and Fungicides

Modern industrial farming methods and the monoculture approach make crops susceptible to pest, and chemical fertilizers make crops deficient in the nutrients that they need. So, if we are going to farm this way, how can we protect these weak, nutrient deficient plants? Of course, we change their genetic makeup and spray them with various kinds of poisons! If insects eat a "Roundup Ready" plant and die, what happens if we eat those same plants?

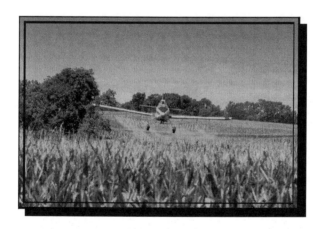

Would you eat poison? Well, you probably do.

2.5.2 Chemical Fertilizers and Depleted Soil

Plants get their nutrients from the soil. If the soil doesn't contain the proper nutrients, the plant has no source for them. Healthy soil is full of organisms that turn dead matter and minerals into nutrients that the plant can use.

Soil that has been treated with chemical fertilizers containing only nitrogen, phosphorus, and potassium (NPK) become depleted of the amazing variety of nutrients that plants need. This means that when we eat those plants we don't get the wonderful variety of nutrients that we should.

2.5.3 GMOs

You may or may not believe in the theory of evolution, but we as humans over thousands of years have changed and adapted right along with our food supply. This is a very slow process. What will the effect of GMOs be on human health? It's too early to tell, but several European countries have already banned the cultivation and sale of GMOs. Do they know something we here in America don't? Probably.

2.5.4 The Dirty Dozen and the Clean Fifteen

Organic produce typically costs more than conventionally grown plants. If you are like most of us, you don't have a lot of extra money to spend, but your health is important. So what can we do?

My suggestion is to buy organic produce for the most important things and conventional for the rest. Many studies have been done to measure the level of pesticides and herbicides in produce. The "Dirty Dozen" were found to contain the highest level of toxins and the "Clean Fifteen" the lowest level. So, whenever possible spend a little extra on the dirty dozen. The list changes a little bit from year to year, but at the time of this writing (2018) here's the list.

The Dirty Dozen include:

1. Strawberries
2. Spinach
3. Nectarines
4. Apples
5. Grapes
6. Peaches
7. Cherries
8. Pears
9. Tomatoes
10. Celery
11. Sweet Bell Peppers
12. Kale

In previous years this list has also included blueberries, collard greens, potatoes, and lettuce.

The Clean 15 include:

1. Avocados
2. Sweet corn
3. Pineapples
4. Cabbage
5. Onions
6. Sweet peas
7. Papayas
8. Asparagus
9. Mangos
10. Eggplant
11. Honeydew Melon
12. Kiwi
13. Cantaloupe

14. Cauliflower
15. Broccoli

In previous years this list has also included watermelon, grapefruit, and sweet potatoes.

2.5.5 Wash Your Produce

Even organic farmers are allowed to use some pesticides, so it's always best to wash your produce. Studies have shown that most commercial "produce cleaners" are no more effective than plain water.

Here's a simple method for washing produce:

1. Fill a large bowl (or your sink) with water.
2. Add a teaspoon of baking soda.
3. Add the veggies.
4. Let soak for a minute or two.
5. Scrub with a brush (except for leafy greens and berries).
6. Rinse.

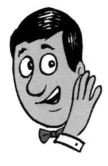

"Of all the living creatures on this planet we are
the only ones that cook our food."

2.6.1 Raw Is Simple and Healthy

A large percentage of my diet is raw food. Eating raw is simple;
you just put it in the blender or juicer, or eat it as is. But more
importantly, raw food is live food. The enzymes and nutrients
are still intact. Cooking destroys virtually 100% of the enzymes
and a high percentage of the vitamins and protein.

Enzymes are kind of mysterious, at least to me. They are
considered the "spark of life" and looked on as "helpers" because
they are catalysts for virtually every function that takes place in
the human body.

Most nutritionists consider 116^0F as the temperature at which
enzymes are destroyed. Therefore soups that are heated until
they are just warm to the touch or foods that are dehydrated are
still considered raw.

Raw foods are naturally high in fiber, moisture, and nutrients.
Therefore they are great for weight loss and preventing chronic
diseases such as heart disease, diabetes, and cancer.

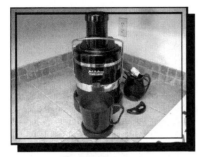

Juicer

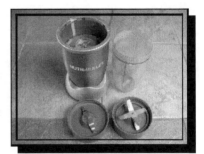

Blender

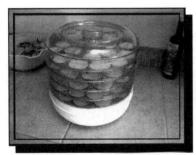

Dehydrator

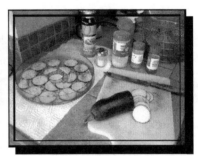

Making Zucchini Chips

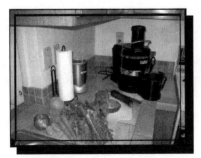

Preparing to Juice

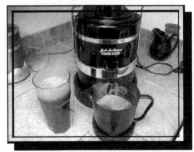

Yum! That Healthy Juice!

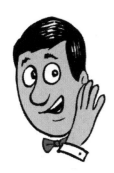

"One of my keys for success is to recognize and embrace the fact that there will be some effort involved. Making a healthy vegetable juice takes some time and effort. Cleaning the juicer afterward is a pain. If you come to dread it, you won't do it! So, don't rush it or wish it was over; just consider it part of the process. As I am cleaning the juicer I think about how great tasting the juice is and all of its health benefits."

2.7.1 Juicing

Juicing is a convenient way to get a powerful shot of nutrients. In one glass of juice you can consume the nutrients from many more fruits and vegetables than you would ever eat at one sitting. Be careful when juicing fruits; not only are you concentrating nutrients, you are also concentrating sugars.

If you were to eat an orange, you would probably eat just one, but if you were to make a large glass of orange juice you would be consuming the sugar from several oranges.

If you add some fruit to vegetable juice it will make it more palatable, but add just a small amount. I especially like to add half of a lemon (skin and all) to a large batch of vegetable juice. Besides having lots of nutrients, it makes the juice taste great!

Is cleaning the juicer a pain? Yes! The trick is to clean it immediately after juicing before the pulp has a chance to dry out and get sticky.

Worried about wasting the pulp? If you have a garden and do composting you can use it there. Also, you can use it to make up a nice vegetable stock to use in the rice cooker or as stock for soups. As shown in Figure 2-11, it's a simple process. After I bring it to a boil, I shut off the heat and let it stand for a few hours to simmer and cool before straining.

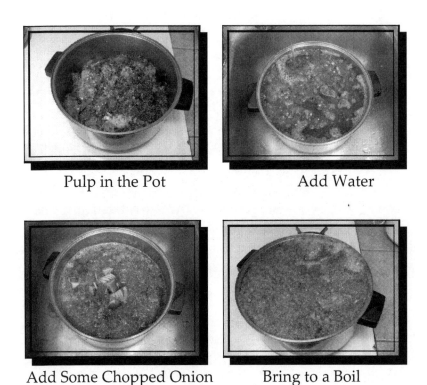

Pulp in the Pot   Add Water

Add Some Chopped Onion   Bring to a Boil

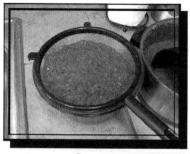
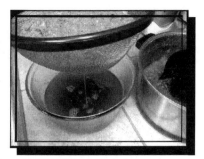

Strain   Final Product

Figure 2-11 Making Vegetable Stock from Juicer Pulp

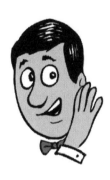

"You may think that buying a juicer and a blender are big expenses, but it's better to spend some money now on reclaiming your health than needing to spend a lot more later on prescription drugs and medical procedures. My heart attack and rehabilitation cost about $100,000.00. Thankfully I am a veteran and the VA paid for most of it. Each year many Americans go bankrupt because of their medical bills."

2.7.2 What to Juice?

I like to include a wide variety of colors in my juices because every plant pigment is a medicine. My juices almost always include some kale, ginger and lemon. Figure 2-12 shows some of the ingredients that I typically include.

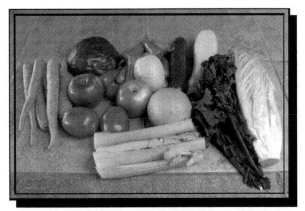

Figure 2-12 Typical Juice Ingredients

2.7.3 Blending

Blending is another easy way to "eat" more fruits and vegetables. With blending you get the whole plant including the pulp, plus you can mix in things that don't juice like bananas, nuts and seeds. Blending is just like eating the whole plant except the blender "chews" it for you. In fact, it chews the food a lot better than you ever could and, by rupturing the cell walls, causes more nutrients to be released. It is recommended that we chew our food thoroughly. If we're lucky we may chew ten times before swallowing. When you run it through a blender it's like chewing it a thousand times!

When I look at the stuff I put in the blender I realize that I would never just sit down and eat all that (especially raw). So, it's a great way to increase the percentage of fruits and vegetables in your diet.

2.7.4 Smoothie Ingredients

As with my juices, I like to mix it up a little with my blender drinks. They usually include a banana, some mixed greens, a date, a fig, a prune, some seeds and nuts, a sprinkle of cinnamon and some turmeric. Figure 2-13 shows some of my typical blender ingredients.

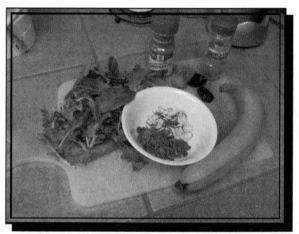

Figure 2-13 Typical Blender Ingredients

2.7.5 Dehydrating

Dehydrating vegetables is a great way to make healthy raw snacks. They are still considered raw because the temperature never gets above 116^0F.

2.8 Juicing Combined with Blending

2.8.1 Some Things Don't Juice Well

Combining juicing and blending has some advantages. Let's say you would like to have some ingredients in your juice that don't have a high enough water content to juice properly like bananas, nuts or seeds. Simple, Just put those things in your blender, pour in the juice and blend. Not rocket science, but something to try. Also, this is a way to add whole fruits to your juice so you don't loose the pulp.

The same idea can be applied if you have a centrifugal juicer that doesn't do well with green leafy vegetables. Juice up stuff like carrots, celery and zucchini, and then use the blender to add the greens.

2.9 Storing Your Produce

I use special bags to store produce. As fruits and vegetables ripen they give off ethylene gas. These bags absorb this gas and extend the life of your produce. Figure 2-14 shows the bags that I use. They are pretty inexpensive and are reusable. As shown in Figure 2-15, if I put produce in a large plastic containers I will simply lay one of these bags over them before putting on the lid.

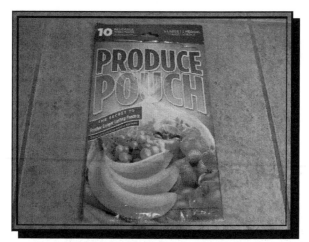

Figure 2-14 Produce Bags

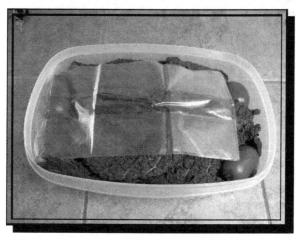

Figure 2-15 Using Bag to Absorb Ethylene Gas

Chapter 3. Foods, Spices, and Gadgets

This may seem obvious, but eating whole foods is a much better way to get nutrients than trying to get them from supplements. With whole foods you get nature's ideal balance of nutrients. Whole foods contain a wide variety of nutrients with just the right amount of each. They work together for maximum absorption, and they come directly from healthy plants, not from a laboratory.

This is not an exhaustive list, just a little something to get you thinking about healthy choices. You should be able to find all of these foods and spices at your local grocery store. Also, you can find a lot more information about their health benefits with a quick search on the Internet. If some are new to you, give them a try. I'm sure you know what most of these foods look like, but I have included little thumbnail pictures just to whet your appetite.

By the time you finish this chapter I hope you will agree that eating a variety of multicolored plants will give you the "symphony of nutrients" that you need for vibrant health.

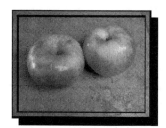

Apples

Apples are rich in antioxidants, flavanoids, and dietary fiber. These nutrients may reduce the risk of developing cancer, hypertension, diabetes, Alzheimer's, Parkinson's, cancer, gallstones, constipation, and heart disease. They also help reduce cholesterol. No wonder they say, "An apple a day keeps the doctor away."

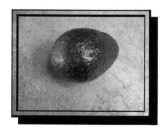

Avocado

Avocados provide a substantial amount of healthy monounsaturated fatty acids. They also have lots of vitamins and minerals.
I use avocado in place of mayo in sandwich's, salads, and any dish where I want to add some richness.

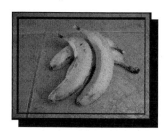

Bananas

Everyone knows that bananas have potassium, but bananas are also high in B-vitamins, magnesium, antioxidants and fiber. Also, bananas contain tryptophan to make you happy, and they reduce swelling, protect against diabetes, and aid in weight loss.

119

Cantaloupe (Musk Melon)

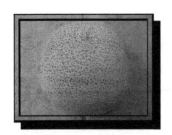

Cantaloupe contains more beta-carotene than most other fruits. Once eaten beta-carotene is either converted to Vitamin A that acts as a powerful antioxidant to help fight free radicals. It also contains vitamin C, folate, fiber, and potassium.

Cherries

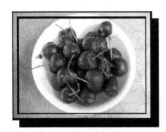

Cherries are rich in antioxidants and contain melatonin, a key chemical to promote sleep. Their anti-inflammatory properties help fight gout and arthritis.

Dates

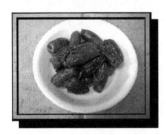

Dates are high in fiber and antioxidants. Also, dates have been shown to improve digestive health, prevent anemia, and promote immune system health.

Grapes

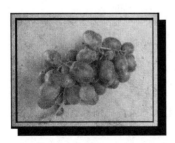

Grapes have anti-inflammatory properties, can help regulate blood pressure, and improve blood flow. Resveratrol, one of the immune-boosting antioxidants found in grapes, is specifically linked to improving blood sugar regulation. Also, grapes may reduce the risk of some cancers.

Honeydew Melon

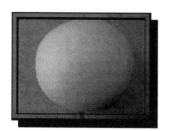

Honeydew melon is rich in fiber that can help lower cholesterol. Also it is rich in calcium, which promotes strong bones and teeth. Studies have shown that it helps reduce hypertension and can boost the immune system.

Lemons

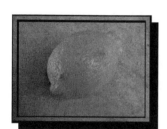

Lemons are high in potassium, vitamin C, and antioxidants. They help to strengthen your immune system, and help keep the blood vessels dilated to reduce hypertension. Besides its health benefits, some lemon in a big glass of vegetable juice makes it taste great!

Oranges

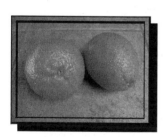

Oranges are rich in citrus limonoids that fight several types of cancer. They also help prevent kidney disease and lower cholesterol. Oranges contain lots of potassium and vitamin C.

Pears

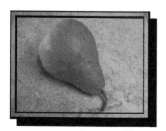

Pears are a great source of dietary fiber that helps improve digestion and aids in weight loss. Like most fruits, pears are rich in antioxidants

121

and vitamins that boost the immune system. Pears contain copper and iron, help to improve circulation and speed healing.

Pineapple

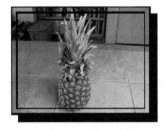

Pineapple is an excellent source of vitamin C, potassium, calcium, and manganese. It also is a great source of dietary fiber, vitamin B-1, vitamin B-6, and folate.

Prunes

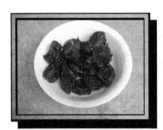

OK, I know what you're thinking! Besides relieving constipation, prunes are a healthy source of vitamin A that is essential for healthy vision. Also, prunes are a powerhouse of antioxidants and potassium. Prunes support heart and bone health.

Raisins

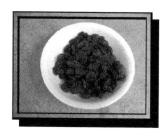

Raisins are rich in fiber for digestive health. They are rich in iron and copper, which help in the treatment of anemia. They are rich in potassium, polyphenols, tannins and antioxidants, help control cholesterol levels and reduce hypertension.

Tomatoes

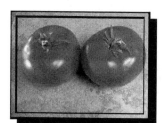

Tomatoes contain large amounts of lycopene, an antioxidant that is highly effective in fighting cancer-causing free radicals. Also, its health benefits include lowering hypertension, improved vision, helping to reduce the oxidative stress of type-2 diabetes, and preventing urinary tract infections.

Watermelon

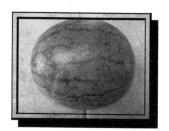

Watermelon has more lycopene than raw tomatoes. It is a heart and immune system healthy fruit. Also, it has anti-inflammatory properties. Watermelon contains beta-carotene, which is good for your skin and eyes. It also contains vitamins A, B-6, C, and potassium. You can eat the seeds and the rind. Just blend them in a smoothie.

Vegetables are so versatile! You can make stir fries, salads, soups, casseroles, and baked vegetables.

As shown in Figure 3-1, the most convenient way I have found to consume them is by juicing or blending them up into a smoothie. Some greens can have a pretty strong taste, so try mixing in a little fruit to sweeten things up.

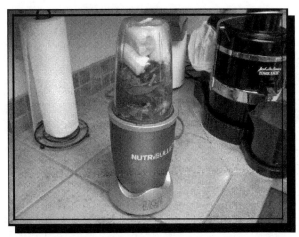

Figure 3-1 Fruit and Vegetable Smoothie

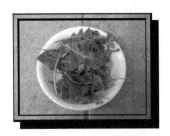

Arugula

Arugula is an excellent detoxifier. It contains vitamin K, for bone health, lots of other vitamins and minerals that boost the immune system, and is an excellent source of carotenoids that help improve eyesight. Arugula also aids in cancer prevention.

124

Beets

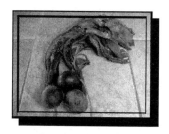

Beets are rich in nitric oxide, which can help open your blood vessels. They are very versatile and can be juiced, baked, or used in stir-fries. Beet greens are an excellent source of beta-carotene, lutein, and zeaxanthin, making them a powerful antioxidant and cancer fighting vegetable. Also, beet greens may slow the effects of dementia.

Bell Peppers

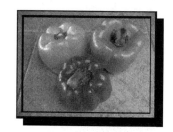

Bell peppers are rich in vitamin C and beta-carotene for immune system health. They are good for eye health, and contain lots of antioxidants for cancer prevention. They help to reduce LDL cholesterol levels, and contain iron to help prevent anemia.

Broccoli

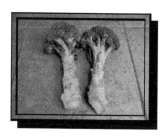

Broccoli is rich in dozens of nutrients. It has cancer fighting and immune system boosting properties. It helps lower cholesterol levels and bolsters heart health. I don't mind buying broccoli with the big stems on them because I run the stems through the juicer.

Brussels Sprouts

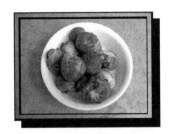

The high fiber content of brussels sprouts helps to lower cholesterol levels. Brussels sprouts contain antioxidants including vitamins C, E, and A, as well as manganese. They have cancer-fighting properties and help promote vascular health. Also, brussels sprouts are high in vitamin K, which is good for bone health.

Cabbage

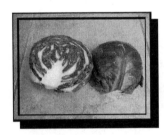

Cabbage helps to reduce chronic inflammation. It is a heart healthy vegetable that may help to lower blood pressure and cholesterol.

Carrots

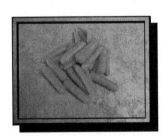

Carrots contain vitamin A and have a host of health benefits including cancer prevention and anti-aging. They are rich in beta-carotene that helps prevent macular degeneration and cataracts. Also, carrots are high in carotenoids that help prevent heart disease.

Cauliflower

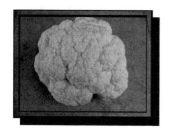

Cauliflower is rich in omega-3 fatty acids and vitamin K, which assist in preventing chronic inflammation. It also is high in fiber and promotes healthy digestion. Cauliflower is high in antioxidants, helps strengthen bones, boost the immune system, and can reduce the risk of developing various forms of cancer.

Celery

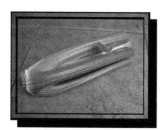

Celery reduces inflammation and helps to regulate the body's alkaline balance. It is high in fiber, to help keep you regular. It also aids in eye health, and the compound butylphthalide helps to reduce bad cholesterol. Celery helps to reduce blood pressure

Cucumbers

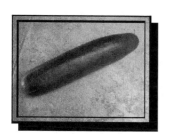

Cucumbers contain an anti-inflammatory flavonol called fisetin that appears to play an important role in brain health. Cucumbers help reduce your risk of cancer. They are high in fiber and contain numerous antioxidants.

Kale

Kale is one of the healthiest and most nutritious foods known. It is loaded with vitamins, minerals, and antioxidants. It can help lower cholesterol levels, and has a number of cancer-fighting compounds. Kale is high in lutein and zeaxanthin, which promote eye health. Also, kale is well known for its ability to promote detoxification.

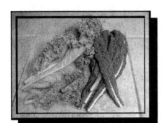

Onions

Onions help prevent colon cancer and boost cardiovascular health. They contain anti-bacterial and anti-microbial compounds that fight against infections. Onions promote bone health and boost the immune system. Also, they help lower blood pressure and fight inflammation.

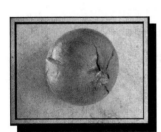

Potatoes

Potatoes are one of the most common food sources on the planet. Their health benefits include their ability to reduce cholesterol levels, boost heart health, prevent cancer, strengthen the immune system, reduce inflammation, and help reduce blood pressure.

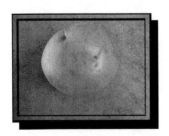

Radish

Radish greens are rich in vitamins C, B-6, and A. They also contain magnesium, iron, calcium, and phosphorus. They help lower cholesterol and boost immunity. Radish root may help prevent certain types of cancer and lower the risk of cardiovascular disease.

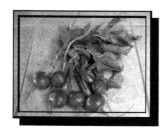

Romaine Lettuce

Iceberg lettuce is pretty low in nutrients, but romaine lettuce is loaded with vitamins, minerals and antioxidants. It is good for weight loss, helps prevent bone loss, helps the skin to heal, boosts heart health, strengthens the digestive tract, lowers the risk of cancer, and improves eye health,

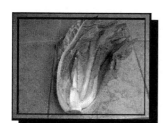

Spinach

Spinach contains many healthy nutrients including CoQ10, lutein, beta-carotene, vitamins C, E and B, omega-3, calcium, magnesium, iron and manganese. Spinach helps to build muscle, improves vision, helps prevent stomach ulcers, helps with weight loss, helps prevent anemia, and helps to relieve arthritis pains.

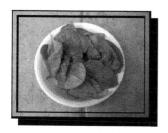

Sweet Corn

Sweet corn is a good source of the antioxidant ferulic acid, which plays a vital role in preventing cancer and inflammation. It also contains B vitamins such as thiamin, niacin, riboflavin and pyridoxine. Corn is a good source of minerals like zinc, magnesium copper, iron and manganese. I usually buy frozen bags of "petite" or "early season" corn. Most nutrition experts agree that frozen corn is just as healthy as fresh picked.

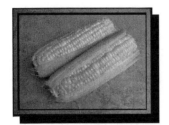

Sweet Potatoes

Sweet potatoes are a good source of the antioxidants vitamins C and A. They help to reduce inflammation, fight against cancer and diabetes, boost heart health, and strengthen the immune system. They help to lower blood pressure because of their potassium content. Also, they are high in fiber, which improves digestion.

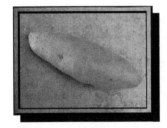

Swiss Chard

Swiss chard is a powerhouse for vitamins and minerals. It has vitamins K, C, E, and B-6, and the minerals magnesium, potassium,

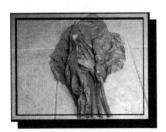

iron, sodium, copper, and manganese. It is also a good source of fiber and antioxidants, so it will help keep you "regular" and fend off various types of cancer.

Squash

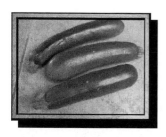

In this category I am grouping zucchini, yellow squash, acorn squash, butternut squash and several others. Squash is high in fiber, and protein, promotes bone and eye health, boost immunity, and helps prevent cancer. It also helps you loose weight, lower blood pressure, and can reduce the risk of heart disease.

Beans

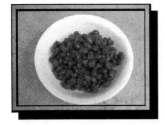

Beans are a staple in my diet (black beans, white beans, black-eyed peas, pinto beans, garbanzo beans, red beans, kidney beans, navy beans). They have lots of protein, fiber, and antioxidants. Also, they promote heart health, reduce the risk of cancer, and are good for gut health. Besides using them in chili dishes and burritos, I often put some in my green smoothies to add a little more protein and fiber. Because I'm lazy I usually buy them in the can, but I dump them in the colander and rinse them before using.

Lentils

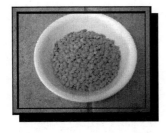

Lentils are rich in many nutrients including protein, fiber, folate, vitamin B-6, thiamin, niacin, riboflavin, vitamin K, iron, magnesium, phosphorus, potassium, zinc, and manganese. Lentils can improve heart health, help stabilize blood sugar, fight cancer, and they are an excellent source of plant protein.

Peanuts

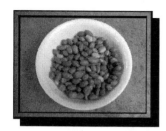

Peanuts contain "good" fat, protein, fiber, niacin, folates, thiamin, copper, manganese, iron, and magnesium. When I was in the Peace Corps in Uganda, I discovered that peanuts are a staple food there. We would grind them up and use them together with tomatoes and spices as a wonderful sauce to go over rice or matoke (a starchy cooking banana).

Peas

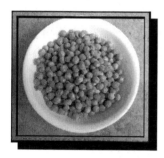

Peas go well in many dishes including soups and fried rice. They are loaded with nutrients that help prevent heart disease, reduce cholesterol, strengthen bones, and boost immune function. I usually buy frozen bags of "petite" or "early season" peas.

3.4 Seeds and Nuts

Seeds and nuts are very healthy foods, but they are high in fat, so they should be used in moderation. They have lots of potassium, magnesium, and other healthy nutrients. It's best to buy them raw. Even though roasting and salting makes them taste better as a snack, the roasting kills all of the enzymes and most of the vitamins.

Almonds

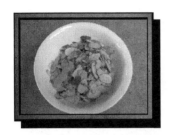

Almonds have a number of health benefits. Thanks to the high concentration of beneficial monounsaturated fats they have the ability to protect heart health. They increase circulation, strengthen the bones, protect the skin, aid in digestion, and help control blood sugar levels.

Cashews

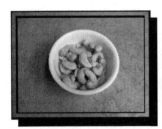

Cashews are high in proanthocyanidins, which help prevent cancer cells from dividing. They are heart healthy and help to lower blood pressure. They promote healthy bones and nerves. Also, the fat in cashews is the healthy kind.

Chia Seeds

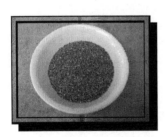

Chia seeds have loads of antioxidants, calcium, manganese, Omega-3 fatty acids, protein and fiber. They help reduce inflammation, are heart healthy, and help strengthen your bones. They are easy to use; just put a teaspoon full in your green smoothies.

Flax Seeds

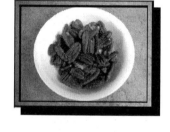

Flax seeds are high in omega-3 fatty acids, fiber, and antioxidants. They help to lower blood pressure and are a good source of protein. I grind them into flax meal with my Nutribullet blender. If not ground into flax meal they tend to just pass right through your system. Flax seeds go great with oatmeal, sprinkled on salads, or mixed in your green smoothies.

Pecans

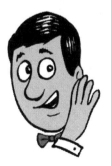

Pecans are high in healthy fat, fiber, manganese, copper, thiamin, magnesium, phosphorus, iron, protein, omega-3 and omega-6 fatty acids. They help boost digestive health, strengthen bones, promote heart health, reduce blood pressure, and are anti-inflammatory.

"Having a slice of pecan pie is not the same as adding some raw pecans to your salad. But, you probably already knew that."

Pistachios

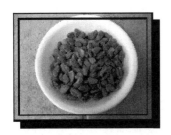

Pistachios are high in protein and fiber, and they have many surprising health benefits. They are a good source of antioxidants, promote healthy gut bacteria, help to lower cholesterol, lower the risk of heart attack, and boost eye health,

Pumpkin Seeds

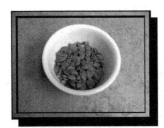

Pumpkin seeds are high in magnesium, zinc, omega-3 fatty acids, fiber, antioxidants, and tryptophan. They help so support heart health, reduce inflammation, boost the immune system, reduce the risk of prostate cancer, and help promote restful sleep.

Sesame Seeds

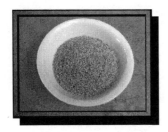

Sesame seeds are a rich source of antioxidants, protein, dietary fiber, and minerals like calcium, iron, potassium, phosphorus, and magnesium. They also contain thiamin, vitamin B-6, folate, zinc, copper, riboflavin, and vitamin E. They help prevent cancer, improve heart health, lower blood pressure, help reduce inflammation, lessen anxiety, and help prevent diabetes.

Sunflower Seeds

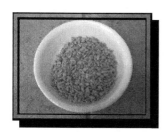

Sunflower seeds are rich in vitamin E, fiber, selenium, copper, and magnesium. They can help lower cholesterol, aid in digestion, help prevent cardiovascular disease, help prevent cancer, and help support bone health.

Walnuts

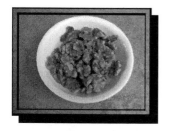

Walnuts are high in omega-3 and omega-6 fatty acids. They also contain other essential minerals such as beta-carotene and lutein. They are a good source of dietary fiber, and are rich in antioxidants. Walnuts are anti-inflammatory, good for heart health, help lower cholesterol, improve sleep, lower blood pressure, and improve brain function.

3.5 Berries

Fresh berries don't keep very well so I usually wash them, and put them in the freezer. Berries go great on oatmeal, in a green salad, or in a smoothie. There are many types of healthy berries. Let me mention just a few of my favorites.

Blackberries

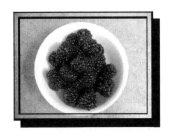

Blackberries are high in vitamins and minerals, fiber, and antioxidants. They have anti-cancer properties, help to improve digestion, are heart healthy, help boost the immune system, improve vision, and support bone health.

Blueberries

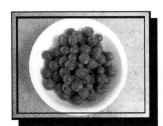

Blueberries contain vitamin C, vitamin K, and manganese. Just like other berries, they are high in antioxidants, are heart healthy, help to prevent cancer, can reduce cholesterol and blood pressure. Wow! No wonder they are considered one of the healthiest berries.

Strawberries

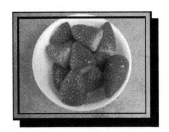

Strawberries are loaded with vitamins, minerals, and antioxidants. They contain vitamins C and K, folate, potassium, manganese, and magnesium. Strawberries help promote eye health, boost immunity, reduce inflammation, reduce the symptoms of arthritis, help lower blood pressure, improve heart health, and have anti-cancer properties.

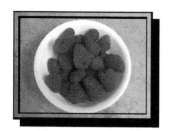

Raspberries

Raspberries are a rich source of vitamins, minerals, and fiber. They help lower the risk of cancer, obesity, and cardiovascular diseases. Also, they help boost the immune system, maintain eye health, and help reduce inflammation.

3.6 Whole Grains

"Whole grains" means not refined or highly processed. In their natural state all grains are whole, consisting of three edible parts - the bran, the germ, and the endosperm.

You will find grains in products like crackers, white bread, and pretzels, but the good nutrients have been refined out of them and chemicals have been added to them.

Today the "staff of life" (wheat) is not the same grain that humans have been eating for thousands of years. It has been sprayed with pesticides and genetically modified to the point where we are seeing a sharp rise in gluten intolerance.

Soy products have been hailed as an excellent animal replacement, but today virtually all soy is a genetically modified organism (GMO).

There are many whole grains that are healthful, but I am pretty boring when it comes to grains. For me it's usually oatmeal or rice.

Brown Rice

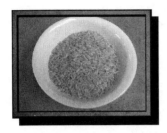

Brown Rice is much better for you than white rice. It has had the hull removed, but still has the nutrient-dense bran and germ. Brown rice is rich in fiber, vitamins, and minerals. It can help control diabetes and obesity, is heart healthy, helps prevent cancer, improves nervous system function, and promotes restful sleep.

Oatmeal

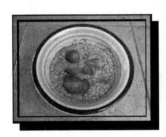

Oatmeal is loaded with fiber and antioxidants. It helps to lower cholesterol and regulate blood sugar, protect against cancer, boost the immune system, promotes sleep, and is gluten free.

3.7 Salad Dressings

Store bought salad dressings often have lots of salt, fat and chemicals that you don't want in your diet. So, why not make your own! Here are a couple of simple and tasty salad dressings.

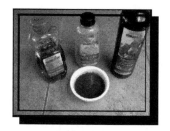

Honey Mustard Dressing

Mix together equal amounts of spicy brown mustard, honey, and water. Then mix in a little bit of balsamic vinegar.

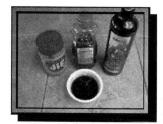

Nut Butter Dressing

Mix together equal amounts of almond butter, honey, and water. Add some balsamic vinegar. Yum! Instead of almond butter you might want to substitute peanut butter or Tahini.

3.8 Herbs and Spices

Herbs are the leaves of plants and **Spices** come from the roots, bark, and seeds. Some plants provide both. The leaves of the cilantro plant are classified as an herb, and the seeds (coriander) are considered a spice.

Many of these spices make excellent replacements for table salt. Salt has a bad reputation because processed foods include so much of it, but salt is essential to our health. The USDA recommends that healthy adults limit their daily intake of sodium to less than 2400 mg (one teaspoon). Those with high blood pressure or heart disease should limit their sodium intake to less than 1500 mg. The average American consumes over 4000 mg per day.

Herbs and spices can be fresh or dried. OK, I'm lazy and pick up most of my spices in the spice section of the grocery store.

Because I'm pretty new to actual cooking (as opposed to warming up a frozen dinner in the microwave) my experience with spices is pretty limited, but the following are a few that I use fairly regularly. They are listed in alphabetical order.

Black Pepper

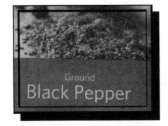

Black pepper is one of those spices that we use to enhance flavor, but we don't usually think about its health benefits. It can aid in weight loss, helps treats asthma and nasal congestion. It also reduces the risk of cancer, heart disease and liver disease. Black pepper is a rich source of minerals like potassium, calcium, magnesium, phosphorus, sodium, and vitamins such as thiamin, riboflavin, niacin, and vitamin B-6.

Cayenne Pepper

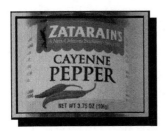

Cayenne contains capsaicin, which can reduce appetite and increase fat burning. It has numerous health benefits such as reducing arteriosclerosis. I love the little bite it adds, so I use it in almost all of my dinners.

Cinnamon

Cinnamon has potent antioxidants. It helps to fight inflammation and has been shown to lower cholesterol and triglycerides in the blood. It has antifungal, antibacterial, and antiviral properties. I like to sprinkle cinnamon on oatmeal and fruits. Also, I like to add a little cinnamon to bean and curry dishes, and sprinkle some in my green smoothies.

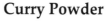

Curry Powder

Curry powder is not just one spice. It is a mixture of spices usually including coriander, turmeric, cumin, and chili peppers. Other ingredients may include ginger, garlic, fennel seed, caraway, cinnamon, clove, mustard, nutmeg, and black pepper. I love curried stir-fry vegetables over brown rice! Curry powder has lots of health benefits including anti-cancer properties, protection against heart disease, and inflammation reduction.

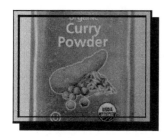

Garlic Powder

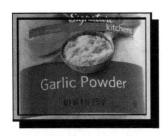

Garlic adds an excellent flavor to soups, chili dishes, veggie pizza, and bean burritos. It helps to reduce LDL cholesterol and lower blood pressure. Most people like to cook with fresh garlic cloves, but I have to admit I usually use garlic powder.

Ginger Root

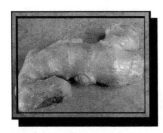

Ginger is a tasty herb to include in juices and smoothies. It has anti-inflammatory, blood pressure lowering, and cholesterol lowering properties.

Himalayan Pink Salt

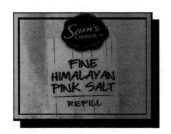

I have substituted Himalayan pink salt for processed salt. It's not just sodium chloride (NaCl). It also has lots of minerals and trace elements. Even so, I try to use just a little bit because I need to continue to work at lowering my blood pressure. Us old guys have to deal with lots of issues.

Turmeric

Turmeric is often used in Asian food, and is the main spice in curry powder. It goes great on roasted veggies and in rice. I also sprinkle some in my green smoothies. Turmeric contains curcumin, a powerful anti-inflammatory and antioxidant. As such, it is used to treat arthritis, joint and stomach pain, Crohn's disease and ulcerative colitis. Curcumin helps to prevent cardiovascular disease by improving endothelial function. The endothelium is the lining of our blood vessels. Studies have shown that turmeric may help prevent certain types of cancer.

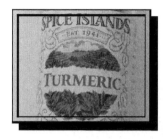

3.9 Foods That Lower Blood Pressure

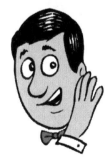

"According to the American Heart Association, 1 in 3 adults has high blood pressure, and 1 in 6 don't even know it!"

This is an important topic to me. My blood pressure has been dangerously high for a long time. My primary care physician has tried several different drugs and combinations of drugs. Just when a new drug appeared to be working I would develop an allergic reaction to it. When your tongue and throat swell up, it is a scary and painful experience!

My eventual goal is to "Let your food be your medicine" as Hippocrates said, and not need to take any drugs.

I have watched several documentaries where obese people went on a plant-based diet and were able to get off all of their meds. Many of them lost weight, but were still obese (we're talking up near 300 lbs), so I think you don't have to reach any certain weight to have normal blood pressure. I think their amazing success was due to their diet. Of course, I want to get down to my ideal weight, but it appears that a person can be overweight and still have normal blood pressure.

Want to reduce your salt intake? If you are eating the SAD diet about 80% of your salt intake comes from processed, prepackaged foods. Just cutting out these highly processed foods will dramatically reduce your salt intake!

The following foods have blood pressure lowering properties. This is just a summary list. For details about each one refer to Sections 3.1 - 3.8 above.

Green leafy vegetables, blueberries, oatmeal, nuts and seeds, garlic, turmeric, basil, cinnamon, black pepper, ginger, pomegranates, apples, bananas, tomatoes, avocado, bell peppers, carrots, beets, sprouts, figs, and potatoes.

The picture below is from my heart catheter test before I went in for triple bypass open-heart surgery. I had severe chest pains and couldn't move very much without becoming completely exhausted. Even if you are the macho type, this is the type of thing you can't just disregard! Believe me, it's not going to just go away. You have to deal with it.

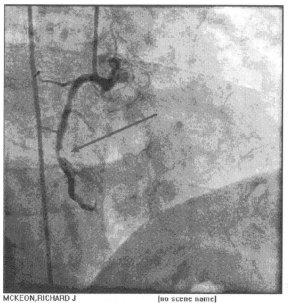

MCKEON,RICHARD J
Carl T. Hayden VAMC
058-34-4488
01/20/1944
Coronary Left Heart Cath

[no scene name]
08/18/2009 2:04:06 PM
RAO: 27. CAUD: 0.4 [Plane A]
Scene: 14
Frame: 40

After my surgery, I used to keep a bottle of nitroglycerin tablets in my nightstand just in case I had chest pains during the night (which I did experience quite often). Everything gets worse at night, and I thought when my heart would race or I had chest pains that I might have another heart attack and die. I'm not afraid of dying, but when you are right there, it is pretty real.

Cholesterol is not an evil molecule. It is necessary for many important metabolic processes, but consuming cholesterol from animal sources is dangerous. Animal proteins can build up in the walls of your arteries, choke off blood flow, and build up plaques. These plaques restrict blood flow to the organs, and when they break off from your artery walls, they create obstructions that block blood flow completely (Can you say heart attack?).

Your liver produces all the cholesterol you need, and plant-based foods have no cholesterol (none, nada, nichts).

Foods that lower cholesterol include oatmeal, whole grains, nuts, citrus fruits, flax seeds, beans, apples, grapes, green leafy vegetables, avocado, and garlic.

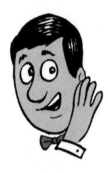

"Does this list look similar to the list of blood pressure lowering foods? Well, here's a little secret. When you use proper nutrition to heal yourself, you don't just heal one thing, you heal EVERYTHING!"

3.11 Foods That Boost Your Immune System

The immune system protects us from harmful invaders like bacteria, viruses, microbes, free radicals, and parasites. Different types of invaders trigger the immune system to produce antibodies. Now, here's an amazing thing; over time your body builds a memory of which antibodies to use for each kind of invader. Is that amazing or what!

Diet and lifestyle choices have a huge effect on how well your immune system functions. Free radicals are molecules from the environment that lack an electron. Once in your body they will steal the missing electron from the atoms of healthy cells. Antioxidants neutralize free radicals by donating an electron of their own. But, even after giving up an electron, the antioxidants remain stable.

Processed foods and alcohol contain lots of free radicals. Also try to avoid toxins from the environment like cigarette smoke, exhaust fumes, and paint fumes. The more free radicals we take in, the harder the immune system needs to work.

Foods high in phytochemicals help boost the immune system. Some of these foods include onions, garlic, kiwi, ginger, carrots, kale, broccoli, brussels sprouts, bell peppers, berries, citrus fruits, mushrooms, apples, sunflower seeds, almonds, oats, and red grapes.

3.12 Foods with Anti-Cancer Properties

We all have cancer cells in our bodies, but usually our immune system keeps them in check. Also, there is mounting evidence that genetics doesn't play as big of a role as we once thought. Here again, diet and lifestyle choices can create an environment in your body that discourages cancer cell growth. Cancer cells love sugar!

Foods that fight cancer are high in fiber and antioxidants. Some of these include garlic, leeks, yellow and green onions, broccoli, brussels sprouts, cauliflower, kale, red cabbage, spinach, beets, zucchini, apples, berries, citrus and brown rice.

If you hear the words, "You've got cancer" that is not an automatic death sentence. Thousands of people are curing themselves with proper lifestyle and nutrition choices.

3.13 Natural Blood Thinners

Most of the time your body's ability to clot is a good thing, but there are times when blood clotting can be dangerous. Foods that help to thin the blood include turmeric, ginger, garlic, cinnamon, whole grains, grapes, raisins, prunes, leafy greens, berries, curry powder, and cayenne pepper.

It's interesting to note that when we consider foods that promote health (lowering blood pressure, boosting your immune system, or fighting cancer) we always get back to a whole-foods, plant-based diet.

3.14 Foods That Reduce Inflammation

Short-term inflammation promotes healing (like when you cut your finger), but chronic inflammation contributes to chronic diseases. Foods high in antioxidants help to lower inflammation. Foods that are highly processes and contain lots of fat and sugar will keep your joints inflamed.

Foods that help reduce inflammation include spinach, blueberries, cherries, avocado, walnuts, papaya, pineapple, green leafy vegetables and turmeric.

3.15 Foods That Stimulate Fat Burning

If you adopt a whole-foods, plant based diet you will naturally start to reach your ideal weight. Foods that are often cited as fat burning include turmeric, tomatoes, kale, broccoli, avocado, brazil nuts, chia seeds, cinnamon, chili peppers, apples, celery, oats, kidney beans, berries, grapefruit and green tea.

3.16 My Meal Plan

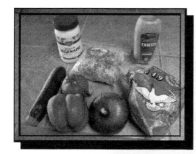
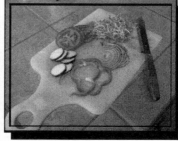
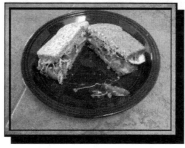

Welcome to the Rick McKeon Culinary School!

OK, that's a little bit tongue in cheek because I know virtually nothing about cooking. Up till now my idea of cooking was to grab a frozen dinner and stick it in the microwave. So, here's an important point.

> If I can make healthy plant-based meals, anybody can!

I'm no expert, but I have been learning a lot from the experts, and I have discovered some easy and delicious meals that I would like to share with you.

I like a high percentage of my meals to be raw. In that case cooking is pretty simple because you don't cook it at all!

In this section I will introduce you to some of my favorite meals. In Appendix A you will find resources with HUNDREDS of recipes for you to try.

3.16.1 Keep It Simple

My meal plan may be too simple for your taste. You can always make your eating plan more interesting and more gourmet than what I present here. In fact, as time goes on I'm sure I will "fancy it up" a bit. But for now these meals are a delicious and nutritious way to get started with the whole-foods, plant-based way of living.

I don't count calories and I eat as much as I want because I am getting enough nutrients to stay satisfied - especially by adding in lots of vegetable juice. You'll notice that I have made the pictures of these meals a little bigger than the other thumbnail images in this book. Why? I'm trying to convince you that healthy eating can be delicious!

3.16.2 Breakfast

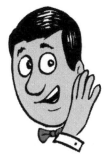

"As far as I am concerned there's nothing wrong with having the same breakfast every day, but I do mix it up a little bit."

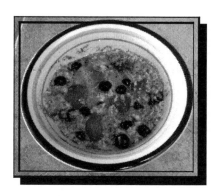

Oatmeal with Berries
I make oatmeal with half oatmeal and half flax meal. Oatmeal is a good source of fiber and helps remove bad cholesterol. Flax meal is loaded with Omega-3 fatty acids. I buy the raw flax seeds and mill them up in my blender. Adding some raisins, cinnamon, and berries makes it even tastier and healthier.

Roasted Tahini and Strawberries on Toasted Ezekiel Bread

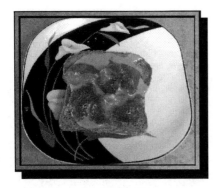

This toast would also be delicious with almond butter or peanut butter and some other fruits like slices of banana. As you can see, the options for toppings are only limited by your imagination! For a real treat, toast the bread up nice and crunchy.

Fruit Bowl

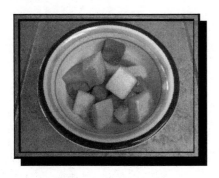

A bowl of your favorite fruits and berries makes a great breakfast. For added nutrition sprinkle on some flax meal, cinnamon, or chopped nuts.

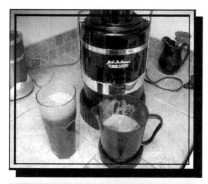

Green Juice
For lunch I usually have a big glass of green juice with plenty of green leafy vegetable. This provides an amazing shot of nutrients!

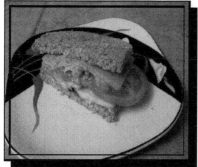

Cucumber and Tomato Sandwich
Of course, the options are endless, but this sandwich has cucumber, tomato, lettuce, brown mustard, soy cheese, and avocado on toasted Ezekiel bread. Yum!

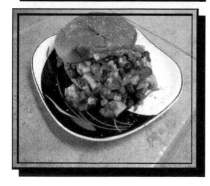

Vegetarian Chili Burger
Have some chili left over from dinner? Make a chiliburger with a whole-wheat bun and some avocado.

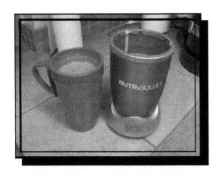

Green Smoothie

Most of my smoothies start out with baby spinach leaves and arugula, a banana and some lemon to sweeten it up. Then I add some nuts and seeds together with a dash of cinnamon..

3.16.4 Dinner

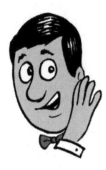

"Dinner doesn't have to be the biggest meal of the day, but if you like to eat a big dinner, try to make it a few hours before bedtime."

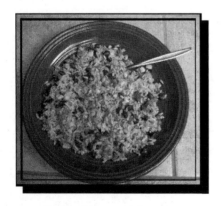

Mixed Vegetables and Brown Rice

This dish is so simple and amazingly delicious! The vegetables can be anything you like. For this dish I used some black beans, frozen corn and peas, and half of an avocado. Plenty of spices and some salsa on top. Yum!

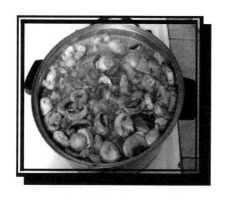

Spicy Vegetable Soup

You can go crazy with this one! Add in all kinds of vegetables and spices. As you can see from the picture, this is a big pot of soup. I typically freeze most of it as individual portions for later use.

In the soup shown above I used an onion, mushrooms, corn, peas, cauliflower, bell pepper, celery, salt, pepper, cayenne, and turmeric. I simply bring it to a boil, turn off the heat, and let it set on the stove for a few hours.

Mushroom Gravy on Whole Wheat Pasta

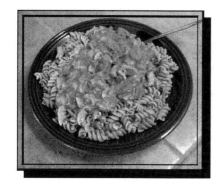

Another simple and tasty dinner. Stir fry the mushrooms and chopped up onion, then add some water and sprinkle with whole-wheat flower to make a thick gravy. I like to season with salt, pepper and garlic powder, and then serve it over whole wheat pasta. Yum!

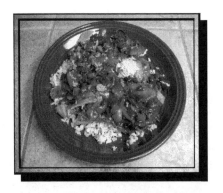

Cabbage, Onions, and Peppers on Brown Rice
Here's another healthy and tasty stir-fry. Of course you can stir in any of your favorite vegetables.

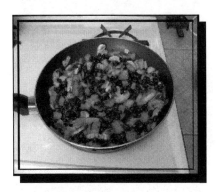

Black Bean Stir-Fry
Stir-fries are so easy and delicious. For this one I used black beans, onions, mushrooms, peppers and spinach. Put it over brown rice or whole-wheat pasta for a delicious and filling dinner.

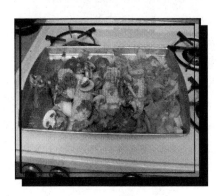

Vegetable Bake
Chop up a bunch of your favorite vegetables, sprinkle with spices, and Bake! This one includes corn, mushrooms, broccoli, bell peppers, and tomatoes.

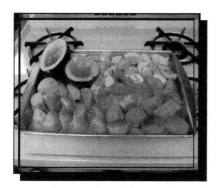

More Vegetable Bake Ideas
Here are a few more ideas for a tasty vegetable bake. This one includes butternut squash, yams, white potatoes, and yellow squash. I put a little honey in the butternut squash.

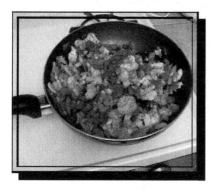

Cauliflower Stir-Fry
The variations are endless! This stir-fry includes cauliflower, onions, mushrooms, and peppers.

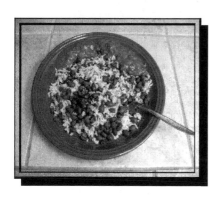

Black Beans and Wild Rice
This one is really simple and tastes great! Just drain and rinse a can of black beans and put it over some wild rice. I sprinkle it with garlic powder, salt and cayenne pepper. A little Salsa on the side and you are good to go!

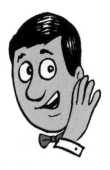

"Because I'm lazy, I will often take the ingredients that I would use in a salad and just throw them in the blender. You are supposed to chew your food several times. Well, with the blender, it's like chewing it a thousand times! Plus you don't have to bother with salad dressing. Of course, making an actual salad adds some nice variety to your eating plan."

Salads can accompany a meal or be a complete meal. Think about your favorite greens, nuts, seeds and fruit. Use your imagination regarding ingredients and dressings. Make it colorful! Here are a few of my favorites.

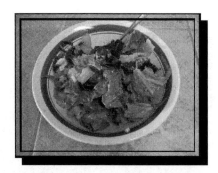

Tomatoes, Cabbage, Lettuce and Peppers
Need salad ideas? Just chop up some of your favorite fruits and vegetables, sprinkle on some seeds and nuts and a little salad dressing.

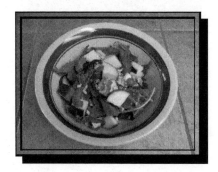

My "Go To" Salad
This salad is simple, healthy, and tasty. Mixed greens, zucchini, and bell peppers with some chopped walnuts sprinkled on top.

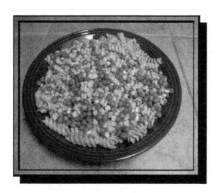

Pasta Salad
What could be easier? Corn, peas, and spices over whole-wheat pasta.

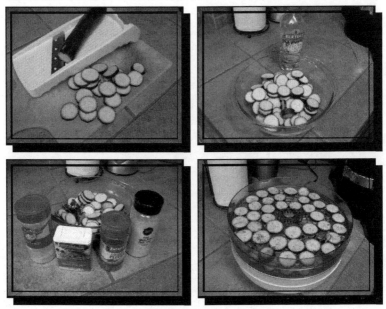

Making Zucchini Chips

Are you in the mood for some potato chips or ice cream? Do your heart a favor and have a healthy snack instead. These snacks are very tasty and satisfying. They are better for you than potato chips, but keep in mind they are snacks, so use moderation.

Avocado

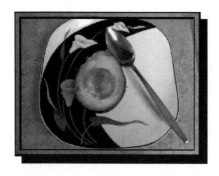

I used to buy avocados and they would go bad before I figured out what to do with them. They go well in salads, but I like to just have a half avocado by itself as a simple and delicious snack. Also, they are a great mayo replacement in sandwiches.

Berries

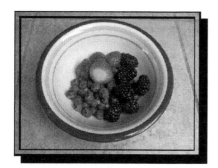

Strawberries, blueberries, or blackberries - you name it! Berries are delicious and loaded with antioxidants. They are high in fiber and vitamins. Enjoy them on their own, add them to smoothies, or put them on your oatmeal.

Black Bean Hummus and Zucchini Slices

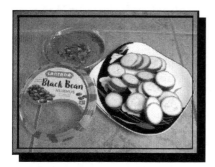

I have to admit that my attempts at making a tasty hummus have been less than stellar, so once in a while I'll treat myself to the store-bought kind. Zucchini slices and organic crackers go great. Also a little salsa does wonders.

Hot Air Popcorn

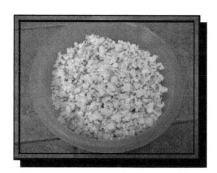

I use an air popper so that I don't have to load it up with butter or oils. For healthy toppings try some of the following: nutritional yeast, balsamic vinegar, cinnamon, cayenne pepper, pureed dates and almonds, or pureed kale and lemon. Get creative with healthy toppings.

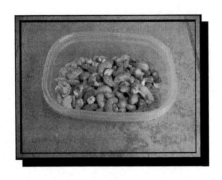

Nuts and Seeds

Nuts and seeds are loaded with protein, healthy fats, and fiber. They also help reduce inflammation. Raw nuts and seeds may not be as appealing as those that are roasted and salted, but they are better for you. Often I will add raw nuts and seeds to a smoothie.

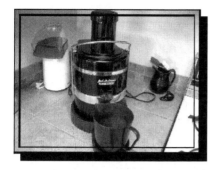

Juicer

There are many juicers on the market today. I have a Jack La Lanne Power Juicer. It's a centrifugal juicer and it is a pain to clean, but it works fine for me.

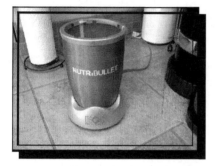

Blender

My blender is a Nutribullet. It has two sets of blades - one for blending, and one for milling. You can turn flax seeds into flax meal in no time.

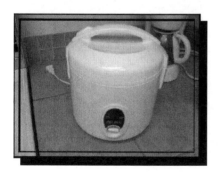

Rice Cooker

My rice cooker is just an inexpensive thing, but it sure makes cooking brown rice simple and easy - just put in rice and water, and it lets you know when the rice is cooked!

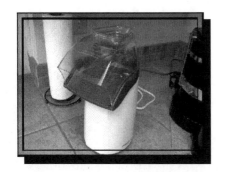

Hot Air Popper

The hot air popper lets me make popcorn without using any oils or butter. If you read the ingredients on microwave popcorn you would be appalled!

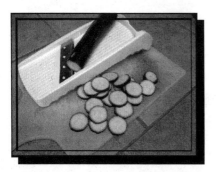

Slicer

Usually I slice things up with a knife, but if I am doing a big batch, I'll get out the slicer. It works great for making zucchini chips. Even if I don't dehydrate them, raw zucchini chips and humus make an excellent, healthy snack.

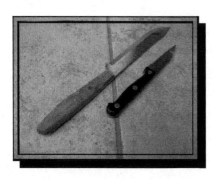

Knives

I have two knives total. A big one and a small one. That's it!

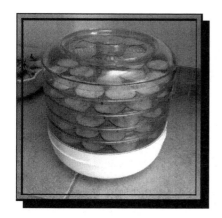

Dehydrator
If you dehydrate produce it
can still be considered raw.
Because the temperature in a
dehydrator is not very high
and the enzymes are not
destroyed

3.18 Simple or Gourmet, It Has to Work for You

The best diet for you is one that you will enjoy and stick with. If you don't like the food or it is too complex to prepare, you won't continue with it. It gets back to the principle that willpower and sheer determination will only last so long.

Chapter 4. How Am I Doing?

There are several health indicators that allow you to track your progress and stay motivated. Here are a few that have worked for me.

4.1 Blood Pressure log

In section 1.1.9 I included my simple blood pressure log. Feel free to photocopy it or use it as a template to create your own log with Microsoft Word or Excel.

4.2 My Baseline Hike

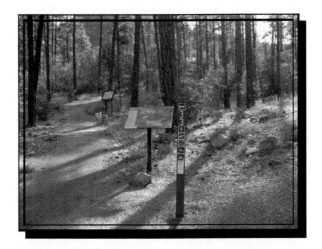

I used to hike a lot until I got sick. Now I am gradually getting back into hiking. To keep it interesting I mix it up and do several different trails up here in the Prescott area, but one hike in particular I call my "baseline hike." It is Trail #33 at Thumb Butte Park. This is a loop hike from the parking lot up to a saddle near the butte. It has a gradual side and a steep side. I like to do this one every so often just to keep track of my progress.

If you take the fork to the right you will be hiking up the gradual side. The fork to the left is a paved trail, but it is much steeper.

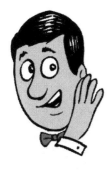

"For video documentaries of several excellent day hikes in Prescott visit my hiking page at: https://www.rickmckeon.com/hiking.html"

I've started hiking up the gradual side with a goal to hike it without stopping. The first time I tried I only got a quarter of the way up and stopped ten times! Anyhow, once my conditioning improves enough so I can hike the gradual side without stopping, I will start hiking the steep side with a goal of hiking it without stopping. I don't know about you, but doing stuff like this helps keep me motivated.

Keeping a diary is another motivator for me. This is not one of those diaries with lots of detailed notes for every day - just significant entries once in a while. Here are a few typical entries. You can see from these few entries that I had my ups and downs. What's the lesson? Don't give up! You will reclaim your health if you just keep on keeping on. I think in my case the slips and setbacks were all part of the learning process.

November 29, 2017, Emergency Room at the VA Hospital

"As I mentioned in the preface, on November 29 I was in the emergency room with some very serious issues. So, here's where the journey begins."

December 6, 2017, Congestion

"I have been sober for just a week and already my congestion is virtually gone! I'm sure it was an allergic reaction to the alcohol"

December 13, 2017, First Hike

"Today I did my first hike in over a year! Just loosing ten pounds was enough to relieve some of the pain in my legs. It wasn't much of a hike, but it's a start!"

December 16, 2017, Blood Pressure

"My blood pressure started dropping right away. Now, after only two weeks it is almost normal (with drugs). How exciting is that!"

December 28, 2017, Good Stats This Morning!

"BP 112/73 (with meds - one day it will be without meds). Weight 250. I was stuck on 252 pounds for three days. From 275 pounds when I started this program one month ago that's a 25-pound weight loss. I'm very encouraged!"

December 28, 2017, Email from My Good Friend Gerard Coard
His emails are an inspiration to me, and I'm sure they will be to you.

"What you said about this program is what I have been thinking. This journey is more than just food and exercise. It's a full transformation.

I was starting to think that I was broken inside. I was questioning my mental/spiritual outlook. It's hard to explain: I love my job, I like who I am, I am optimistic and love life and all people. But! I felt something was missing. I felt a sense of loss after I saw the weight coming back on, yet I was powerless to turn myself around. It just was not happening. I became an expert at finding excuses not to put on my sneakers and walk outside. I hated that I knew so much about eating well, and loved the feeling I got when I climbed South Mountain, but

171

was almost powerless to do anything. Some might call that depression, but I will not go there.

I can't wait to have a month of this new routine behind me. I have wanted this change so badly. Life is wonderful!"

December 30, 2017 Email from Gerard

"There is something so cathartic about having a purpose and an intent, and taking the first step. I have been juicing celery first thing every morning for the last few days, and that has brought my mind back to focusing on healthy living. Would you believe that I have not had any alcohol, or coffee, or even meat, for the last few days? Instead I have been drinking turmeric tea, and eating all kinds of vegetables and loving it. I just don't want to undo the good I have been doing for my body these last few days, and that is pointing me in the right direction.

I noticed too that watching FMTV is like having a companion guide in the house. I have watched so many programs and have learned so much, that I am almost driven to be an activist."

January 1, 2018, Happy New Year!

"December 2017 was a good month. I lost 25 pounds. My blood pressure went from extremely high to normal (still taking BP meds). I am regaining strength in my left arm, and the vision in my right eye is almost back to normal. The pain in my legs is gone, so I am back to regular hiking. The congestion and coughing fits are gone. I'm sleeping much better and getting up earlier. I feel much more energetic and am spending more time on my various projects (including this book). I saved about $400 by not buying a 12-pack of beer every day. All that in one month! Wow, this program is working!"

January 2, 2018, An Exciting Milestone

"Today I 'broke into' the 240's. When I saw 249 on the scale I was very pleased. I started this journey at 275 pounds and have a goal of getting down to 225 pounds, so I still have a long way to go. But this is an exciting milestone. One of the motivators that I mention in Section 1.3.9 is Enjoy Every Victory, Even the Small Ones. Well, I am really enjoying this small victory!"

January 3, 2018, Doctor Visit and Stress Test

"Had a stress test today. I only made it two minutes, but that was long enough for them to get the readings they needed. They also took ultrasound videos of the heart, and the doctor said it looks good with no blockages. What a relief!"

January 10, 2018, Consult with the Oncologist

"This was a scary visit! Based on my blood chemistry she thinks I may have bone marrow cancer. I am scheduled for a CAT scan next month and she sent me down for another blood draw. They took 10 vials of blood!
Some of the bad numbers have come down quite a bit this last month, so I'm hoping that my new diet and exercise program have made the difference. If so, I should be able to bring all the numbers back to normal as I continue to eat a plant-based diet, exercise, and loose weight. In any case, I am going the natural route and will not submit to chemotherapy or radiation treatments!"

January 12, 2018, Excellent Hike Today!

"Today was a perfect day for hiking - bright blue skis and a cool breeze. This is the first day since I've been back hiking that I felt strong even

on the uphill sections. I'm sure that the weight loss and Vegan diet are improving my health and strength. Just a month ago I would struggle with the slightest incline. Now I can push right through it!"

January 14, 2018, Sleep

"This is very strange. I slept the entire night last night. I can't remember the last time I have slept like that. Usually I am awake every hour and sometimes for hours at a time. Last night I put some Aspercreme on my feet around 1:30 because I still have quite a bit of neuropathy, but outside of that I was asleep the whole night! It must be another benefit of this incredible program!"

January 16, 2018, Bummer!

"My weight has been at 243 lbs for a couple of days. This morning I was hoping it would be 242, but it was 244 lbs! So, what's the lesson? Even if you are eating healthy foods, if you eat too much you will gain weight."

January 24, 2018, A Slip and Recovery

"On January 20th I 'fell off the wagon' and drank a 12-pack of beer and ate a double cheeseburger - how crazy is that! Boy, did I pay the price. My weight and blood pressure immediately shot up. It has taken four days to get back to where I was a week ago. Lesson? When I stay motivated it's easy to stick with the program. If I go back to my old ways, things will fall apart immediately!"

April 12, 2018, Amazing changes!

"Today I had a follow up visit with my primary care physician at the VA, Tim McGhee. He was amazed at the improvements in my numbers. Last time my labs indicated that I was in Stage 3 kidney failure. He said that if I would have kept going the way I was the next thing would be dialysis, and after that death. Well, my numbers at this time are normal!"

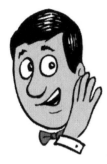

"The big gap in this diary represents several months with lots of ups and downs, but I'm not giving up!"

September 1, 2018, Here We Go Again!

"Like the old song 'Back in the Saddle Again' I am back on the program again'
A few months ago I had an allergic reaction to the Lisinopril, so Tim gave me a 30-day supply of Amlodipine. It worked great for a while and then I had an allergic reaction to it too. This is a serious situation! My goal is to get off all prescription drugs, but I need to keep the blood pressure out of the danger zone until then.

Last Sunday I broke a crown off and went to the dentist Monday morning. She almost didn't treat me because my blood pressure was 197/97. Very dangerous territory! I got back on the meds and the Vegan program, and both my blood pressure and weight started dropping. Many of you reading this are probably asking 'Will he ever get it together?' Well, that's the goal."

October 26, 2018, Another Allergic Reaction!

"We have been trying all kinds of blood pressure meds without success. Tim prescribed another one for me to try. It worked great yesterday, but, as shown in Figure 4-1, today I had a severe allergic reaction - very scary. Looks like I may have to lower my blood pressure using diet and lifestyle changes only."

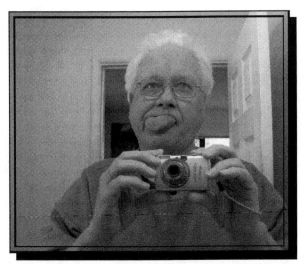

Figure 4-1 Another Allergic Reaction

November 20, 2018, Good News Regarding My Blood Pressure!

"I saw my primary care physician at the VA today. He was pleased with my progress and said, 'Keep on doing what you're doing.' My BP meds haven't changed, but my blood pressure is coming down. This is proof that eating the foods listed in Section 3.9 is working!"

December 10, 2018, The Plant-Based Diet Is Working!

"Had visit with my primary care physician today. All of my blood and urine numbers are in the normal range! I have lost 40 pounds from my high earlier this year, and my blood pressure is almost normal. I am taking just a little bit of Metoprolol, but I expect to be off it in the next couple of months."

January 16, 2019, Neuropathy

"Last night was the first time I made it through the night without having to use pain relief cream on my feet for the neuropathy. They still bothered me quite a bit, but I didn't have to resort to pain relief cream. I'm hoping this is a good sign."

February 7, 2019, Wow! I broke 230 Pounds!

"I'm so pleased! This morning my scales read 228 lbs. I haven't been below 230 lbs in MANY years."

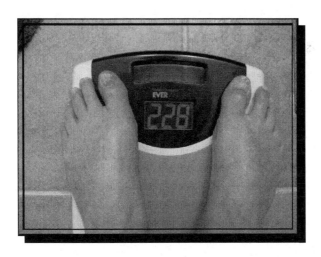

Chapter 5. Wow! Emotional Healing Too?

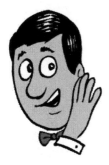

"I didn't even think to include a chapter like this until I was well into the program. Then one morning I woke up and realized that I was experiencing not just physical healing, but emotional healing too!"

5.1.1 A Complete Life Change

This is a strange and unexpected turn of events. I always considered this program to be a "complete life change" but I never thought about emotional healing until I started to experience it.

5.2 What Is Emotional Healing?

So, what is emotional healing and how do you know it's happening to you?

Also, what is spiritual healing and is there a connection between your physical, emotional and spiritual health? I am becoming convinced that these are three different components of a complete person.

In the Preface of this book I stressed that I am not a medical doctor, and I am not offering medical advise. Well, I have to admit here that I am not a trained psychologist either. All I can do is tell you about what is happening to me. My attitude about who and what I am has changed. Emotional healing for me has exhibited itself in several ways.

5.2.1 From Inferiority Complex to Self Worth

Some people seem to have been born with a healthy self worth. In fact, some people seem to have an inflated ego and unrealistic sense of self worth.

I have always been the opposite of that. I don't know if it was genetics or upbringing (in the 1950's), but I have always had an inferiority complex. I don't know where it came from, but I have always felt that I didn't measure up. Therefore I was always looking for approval from others. This feeling has held me back in many situations including personal relationships and in my career. If you feel you aren't deserving of respect, you won't treat yourself with respect and kindness.

I think this was the attitude that led to my recent health issues. I didn't believe that I was worthy of radiant health. After all, I was getting old and living an unhealthy lifestyle. Of course I was sick; that was what I deserved!

Part of my emotional healing was coming to realize that I do have value, and I do have something to give. I'm hoping the lessons from this book will be of value to many. By eating a healthy plant-based diet you are telling yourself with every meal that you have self worth and you do have things of value to share with others.

A healthy self worth is not arrogance or feeling that you are better than others. It is simply acknowledging that you do have value and something to give. Now, I am starting to treat myself with kindness, and as if I mattered.

5.2.2 From Ambiguity to Clarity of Purpose

Can a person live with ambiguity? Can a person go on year after year living a life that is in opposition to his or her own beliefs? Well, I did. I think alcoholics like me do that all the time.

Most people reading this book are probably not alcoholic, but I bet many have ambiguities in their lives. Is there something you want to do, but just can't bring yourself to do it? Conversely, is there something you want to stop doing (smoking, overeating, procrastinating, etc.), but just can't?

That state of affairs has to set up internal conflict and guilt. Now, with improving health and sobriety, I live with the joy that comes from clarity of purpose and lack of internal conflict. More and more I do things right away instead of putting them off and having them hanging over my head for days or weeks. Emotional healing? You bet!

5.2.3 Gratitude and Joy

I may be hiking along a mountain trail or simply wake up in the middle of the night and, all of a sudden, I will be filled with an overwhelming sense of joy and gratitude. Where does that come from? I'm not discounting a spiritual component, but I think it's a combination of things that are part of the physical and emotional healing that I am experiencing.

I certainly know what the joy and excitement of a beer buzz is like. I have experienced that many times, but this joy runs deeper and doesn't come with a price. This joy is healthy and motivating.

5.3 Life Is More Than Just Being Alive!

Just being alive is good, but there is more to it than that. Having a sense of purpose and hope for the future makes for a rich and enjoyable life.

5.3.1 Joy Is More Than a Beer Buzz

This may sound like hype, but it is true. I wake up each morning with new creative ideas. I used to think the only way to enjoy playing blues on the guitar or to enjoy fascinating ideas about patterns in nature was to have a few beers in me. But now I have a greater sense of clarity and am more excited than ever to explore new things and think interesting thoughts. For me sobriety (you can substitute "food addiction" if that is your thing) is only one facet of healthy living.

A clean plant-based diet combined with physical exercise has created a healthy environment not just for my body, but also for my mind! I used to think the phrase "life is more than just being alive" was just some psychological double talk, but I'm starting to understand what it means.

Good health is more than just the absence of pain and disease; it is energy, enthusiasm, and joy.

Finally being able to purchase that special thing (new car, cloths, etc.) that you have been longing for may make you happy for a while, but it won't bring permanent happiness. Focusing on your own needs doesn't bring happiness.

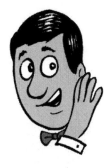

"This may seem counterintuitive, but focusing on the happiness of others and trying to help them enjoy life instead of focusing on yourself will bring you happiness."

We each have unique personalities, talents, and interests, but no matter who you are, you have something special that you can give to others. It might be something as simple as giving a sincere compliment that will light up someone's day. Serving others will bring you joy. Having a purpose to bring joy into other people's lives will bring you permanent happiness.

Chapter 6. The "E" Word

6.1 It Has to Work for You

The benefits or regular exercise include:

1. Lower blood pressure
2. Improved heart health
3. Decreased feelings of depression
4. Weight loss
5. Improved muscle and bone health
6. Increased energy level
7. Increased insulin sensitivity
8. Improved brain function
9. Improved quality of sleep
10. Reduced chronic pain

Everybody is different when it comes to exercise. Factors that might affect your choice of exercise include your age, strength, current physical condition, time availability, and especially what you like.

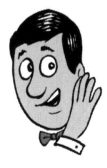

"Drinking beer and watching football on TV does not qualify as exercise!"

That may sound silly, but we can sometimes fool ourselves into thinking that if we watch sports, talk about sports, hang out with sports-minded people, know all the stats, etc. that we are somehow into sports. Not true, you have to get out there and do it yourself.

There is not one "best" form of exercise. The best exercise for you is the one that you enjoy doing and will be able to continue. If it hurts or you dread it, you won't be doing it long! So, choose something you will enjoy and be able to stick with. As your health improves your choice may change, but it is important to just pick something and get started.

You may enjoy yoga, mountain biking, running or kayaking. The list is endless. Just pick something and get moving.

6.2 Hiking

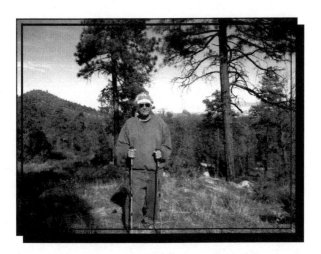

For me hiking is the most pleasurable form of exercise. Living in Prescott, Arizona, I am surrounded by beautiful Ponderosa Pine forests in the Bradshaw and Sierra Prieta mountains with hundreds of wonderful hiking trails. Walking is not as hard on your joints as other high-intensity forms of exercise, and walking just 30 minutes a day can reduce your risk of many common lifestyle diseases including diabetes, heart disease, cancer, and even depression. You don't need to buy into the "No pain, no gain" philosophy. Just go out and take a pleasant walk.

Hiking is free. You don't have to pay for an expensive gym membership that you probably won't even use. Walking helps to boost your immune system.

If you are into jogging, weight training, mountain biking, boxing, or kayaking, that's great! But for me, just taking a hike does the trick. This low-intensity exercise provides all of the health benefits I need.

Now, I'm not a doctor, but I have the distinct impression that with each step, you are giving yourself a nice foot massage - squeezing those feet and increasing blood flow. You could buy an expensive foot massage machine, but simply taking a walk does the same thing. Plus, it gets you out into the fresh air and sunshine (vitamin D) and you have a chance to commune with nature. It's amazing how something as simple as taking a walk can have so many health benefits!

While I'm out on my hikes it's not just about exercise and fresh air. A hike in the forest is a pleasant time for meditation, prayer, and noticing the beauty of the natural world. I get most of my inspired ideas while out hiking.

When I first started back to hiking I was obese and way out of shape, plus I had pretty severe neuropathy in my feet. I was the slowest one on the trail. Everyone was passing me. Now, I've never been competitive, but that was ridiculous! I was not just slower than everyone else; I was WAY slower than everyone else.

I didn't push myself to go faster. I always just hike at a pace that is comfortable. After only a few weeks an amazing thing started to happen; I just naturally wanted to pick up the pace. It felt good to walk faster. Also, I just naturally wanted to include more uphill sections in each hike. That's got to be a good sign.

What if you have trouble just walking? You can still exercise in a pool or sitting in a chair. Anything to get you moving!

Chapter 7. My "Big Adventure"

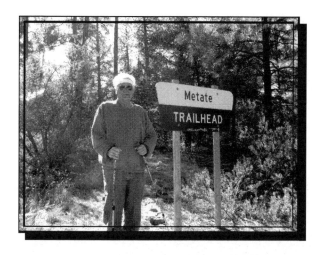

For my big adventure I decided I would try to hike up to Blair Pass on Granite Mountain. I have done this hike many times in the past, but since my recent health issues I haven't been able to hike that far. Actually, I haven't been able to hardly walk at all. So, doing this hike represents a major breakthrough for me. I chose a beautiful spring day and gave it a shot. What a wonderful hike!

7.1 Sore Feet and Satisfaction

The hike went really well. I ended up with sore feet, but also a great deal of satisfaction. This beautiful hike is the furthest I have walked in several years! I had a great time and met some interesting people along the way. After this adventure I am not placing any limits on what is possible. I may even be able to do some backpacking up in the Sierra Nevada Mountains again. Who knows?

Trail 361 up to Blair Pass is a beautiful shaded path along a creek. There was a nice cool breeze blowing, and everything was perfect! It was one of those "magic moments" and I was floating along the trail knowing what a gift it was to be able to do this hike. Many times the trail was almost like a tunnel with the trees wrapped above you. Here are a few pictures I shot along the way.

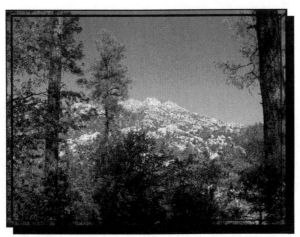

Figure 7-1 Granite Mountain from the Parking Lot

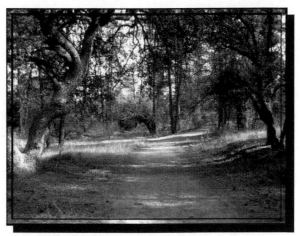

Figure 7-2 Under the Canopy

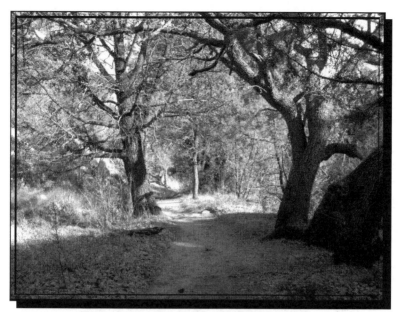

Figure 7-3 Beautiful Juniper Trees

Chapter 8. Fifteen Months Later

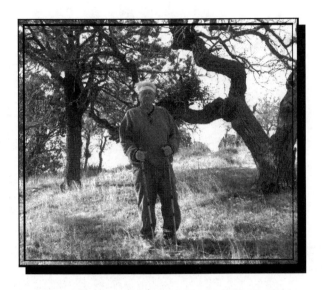

8.1 My Life Today

8.1.1 A Bumpy Road

As with most things that I do, I got off to a rough start and had relapses along the way, but I kept getting back on the program and have made some permanent changes in my health, diet, and lifestyle.

Today, a little over a year after that dreadful day in the emergency room, my life is completely different! Some of the changes I have been able to make include:

1. My blood pressure is down in the normal range, and I have been able to eliminate all prescription medications. This is a major triumph because I have had hypertension for the last 30 years!

2. The strength and feeling in my left arm have returned to normal.
3. The vision in my right eye is normal - no more blind spot.
4. My blood chemistry is normal. I do not have kidney failure, diabetes, or cancer.
5. I have gone from being barely able to walk to completing a hike up to the Blair Pass on Granite Mountain.
6. I have lost 50 pounds.
7. My skin rashes and extreme itching are gone. Why? I'm not sure, but some type of autoimmune disease probably caused them.
8. I sleep better, wake up earlier, wake up refreshed, and wake up with gratitude.
9. I am more ambitious and more productive.
10. My mind is clearer and I have many more creative ideas.
11. I feel that I have more control in my life and I am not just a victim of circumstances. I do things right away instead of putting them off, and I take responsibility for my own actions. That may seem like normal behavior to you, but it certainly wasn't for me.
12. My attitude has changed from one of low self-esteem and the belief that I deserve to be sick to one of self-worth. Today I have the desire to treat myself with love and respect.
13. Because of the mercy and forgiveness God has shown me, I want to show that same mercy to others. I want to encourage others whenever I can.

8.2 The Journey Continues

So many wonderful things have happened during the last fifteen months because of a change in attitude and a few simple lifestyle changes, but the journey continues.

8.2.1 Future Goals

Here are some of my goals for the future:

1. My current weight is 225 lbs. and I have set a new target of 200 lbs. (maybe even lower once I get there). I hope to achieve this weight goal by the end of 2019, and maintain it thereafter.
2. I would like to hike to the summit of Granite Mountain and backpack in the Grand Canyon again.
3. Years ago I did several backpacking trips in the Sierra Nevada Mountains of California. Many of my fondest memories are from those trips. I hope to do at least a two-week hiking trip up there and find myself again.
4. The neuropathy in my feet is almost gone, but this may take a while. I look forward to the day when it is completely gone.
5. I hope to continue this exciting adventure and to share what I have learned with others. I have started a "Health and Wellness" page on my website at https://www.rickmckeon.com/

I hope you have enjoyed reading about my journey and have found something of value here. I would love to hear from you. Please send me an email at rmckeon5@gmail.com

If I had not made the changes described in this book, I would probably be dead by now. This journey wasn't always easy, but I made the changes necessary to pull myself back from the brink and start on an amazing health journey.

I've said it before, but this is the thought I would like to leave with you. You need to take responsibility for your own health. You can't just go to a medical professional, give him some money, and say, "Fix me."

I urge you to follow the guidelines set out in this book and design a program that works for you. You will start to see positive results right away, and over time you will reclaim your health!

Appendix A: Resources

We are fortunate today to have many interesting and motivational sources of information available to us. Not all of these resources will say exactly the same thing, but if you study them all you will find the information that is right for you.

Keep in mind that this is YOUR PROGRAM. It has to work for you in terms of your schedule, your preferences, and your personality. You need to put together a program that you will like and that you can live with for the rest of your life.

A.1 Experts to Follow

I am not an expert, but I have learned from those who are. More than ever before, today there are many experts in the field of nutrition and health who are willing to share their knowledge and experience. Most of the people I am going to mention here are doctors (M.D.) who were classically trained in the pharmaceutical approach to medicine, but who eventually discovered the relationship between diet, lifestyle, and health. There are many more experts making valuable contributions than I list here, but these are a few of my favorites.

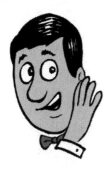

"All of these experts emphasize the fact that the human body has amazing self healing abilities. All we have to do is create an environment within our bodies that will allow it to heal itself! This means introducing healthy micronutrients and eliminating the toxins. How simple is that!"

Adams, Mike

Mike Adams, the "Health Ranger," is an outspoken consumer health advocate, award-winning investigative journalist, Internet activist and science lab director. He is the founder and editor of NaturalNews.com, the Internet's most-trafficked natural health news website. His website address is http://www.healthranger.com/

Barnard, Neal. M.D.

Neal D. Barnard, M.D., F.A.C.C., is an author, clinical researcher, and founding president of the Physicians Committee for Responsible Medicine (PCRM). Barnard serves as an Adjunct Associate Professor of Medicine at the George Washington University School of Medicine. He founded the Barnard Medical Center in 2015 as part of PCRM, and it opened in 2016 with him as president. The center provides primary care and emphasizes diet and preventative medicine. For more information visit https://www.pcrm.org/about-us/staff/neal-barnard-md-facc

Bisci, Fred, Ph.D.

Fred Bisci is a nutritional counselor and raw food pioneer. His program is called *Your Healthy Journey*. This program integrates raw organic plant food combinations with a moderate amount of cooked portions. His website is located at https://www.yourhealthyjourney.org/

Calabrese, Karyn

Karyn Calabrese is a raw food chef and founder of *Karyn's Fresh Corner*. Her program of healthy eating and regular detoxification has advocates raving about its benefits. Her website address is
https://www.karynraw.com/

Campbell, T. Colin, Ph. D.

Colin Campbell is professor of Nutritional Biochemestry at Cornell University. He is the author of over 300 research papers and three books, *The China Study*, *Whole*, and *The Low-Carb Fraud*. He has been featured in several documentary films about the effect of nutrition on long-term health. His website address is https://www.nutritionstudies.org/

Carr, Kris

Kris Carr is a multiple New York Times best-selling author, wellness activist and cancer survivor. She is the subject and director of the documentary *Crazy Sexy Cancer*. Kris is also a member of Oprah's SuperSoul 100, recognizing the most influential thought-leaders today and was named a "new role model" by The New York Times. Her website address is
https://www.kriscarr.com/

Colquhoun, James and Laurentine

James Colquhoun and Laurentine ten Bosch are nutritional consultants and filmmakers. Motivated by a chronic illness in their own family, they created the documentary *Food Matters*. It has become an internationally acclaimed documentary about the medical and healthcare industries. Their FMTV website has gone on to become a leading resource in the natural health world. Their website address is https://www.fmtv.com/

Cousens, Gabriel, M.D.

Gabriel Cousens functions as a holistic physician, homeopath, psychiatrist, and family therapist. In addition, he's a world leading diabetes researcher, ecological leader, spiritual master, founder and director of the *Tree of Life Foundation* and *Tree of Life Center US*. His website address is http://www.treeoflifecenterus.com/

Cross, Joe,

Joe Cross is an Australian entrepreneur, author, filmmaker, and wellness advocate. He is most known for his documentary *Fat, Sick & Nearly Dead* in which he tells the story of his 60-day juice fast. He is the founder and CEO of *Reboot with Joe*, a health and lifestyle brand. His website address is https://www.rebootwithjoe.com/

Esselstyn, Caldwell B., M.D.

Dr. Esselstyn is a physician, author and former Olympic rowing champion. He is the author of *Prevent and Reverse Heart Disease* in which he demonstrates the benefits of a whole-foods, plant-based diet. His website address is http://www.dresselstyn.com/

Esselstyn, Rip

Rip is the son of doctor Caldwell Esselstyn. For ten years he was a very successful professional athlete, so you know the diet and lifestyle that he learned from his father works. He is the author of *The Engine 2 Diet, Plant-Strong,* and *The Engine 2 Seven-Day Rescue Diet*. He is known as an advocate of a whole food, plant-based diet and he also provides some health and wellness retreats. His website address is https://www.engine2diet.com/

Fuhrman, Joel, M.D.

Joel Fuhrman uses a nutrition-based approach to obesity and chronic disease that he refers to as a "nutritarian" diet. He has written several books and has appeared in several health and wellness documentaries. His website address is https://www.drfuhrman.com/

Gabriel, John

Jon Gabriel attended the Wharton School at the University of Pennsylvania. While there, he pursued extensive coursework in biochemistry and performed research for the internationally recognized biochemist Dr. Jose Rabinowitz. After loosing 220 pounds, he developed *The Gabriel Method* for weight loss. You can find him at
https://www.facebook.com/Gabriel.Method

Greger, Michael, M.D.

Michael Herschel Greger is a physician, author, and professional speaker on public health issues, particularly the benefits of a whole-food, plant-based diet and the harms of eating animal products. His website address is https://www.nutritionfacts.org/

Klaper, Michael, M.D.

Dr. Michael Klaper, is a gifted clinician, internationally recognized teacher, and sought-after speaker on diet and health. He has practiced medicine for more than 40 years and is a leading educator in applied plant-based nutrition and integrative medicine. His website address is https://www.doctorklaper.com/

McDougall, John A., M.D.

John A. McDougall, M.D. has been studying, writing, and speaking out about the effects of nutrition on disease for over 30 years. He and his wife Mary believe that people should look and feel great for a lifetime. Their website address is https://www.drmcdougall.com/

Ornish, Dean, M.D.

Doctor Ornish is a clinical professor of medicine at U.C. San Francisco and president of the Preventive Medicine Research Institute. For the last forty years he has directed a series of randomized control trials showing how powerful just a few simple changes in diet and life style can be. Throughout these trials he has demonstrated that these changes can prevent and even reverse most chronic illnesses like diabetes, coronary artery disease, and hypertension. His website address is http://www.deanornish.com/

Popper, Pamela, PhD, ND.

Dr. Pam Popper is a naturopath, an internationally recognized expert on nutrition, medicine and health, and the Executive Director of The Wellness Forum. Her website address is https://www.drpampopper.com/

Robbins, John

John's work has been the subject of cover stories and feature articles in The San Francisco Chronicle, The Los Angeles Times, Chicago Life, The Washington Post, The New York Times, The Philadelphia Inquirer, and many of the nation's other major newspapers and magazines. His life and work have also been featured in an hour long PBS special titled *Diet For A New America*.

The only son of the founder of the Baskin-Robbins ice cream empire, John Robbins was groomed to follow in his father's footsteps, but chose to walk away from Baskin-Robbins and the immense wealth it represented to pursue what he calls "The dream of a society that is truly healthy, practicing a wise and compassionate stewardship of a balanced ecosystem." His website address is https://www.johnrobbins.info/

A.2 Video Documentaries

For videos I typically go to:

1. FMTV (Subscription but well worth it).
2. Netflix: Everybody knows Netflix for entertainment, but they do have several excellent health documentaries. (Subscription).
3. YouTube (Free).

There are lots of documentaries available on health and wellness. Here are a few of my favorites. A quick Internet search will yield more information about each of these documentaries.

100 Days in the Raw (2014)
Six friends try the raw Vegan lifestyle for 100 days with surprising results. For more information visit:

https://www.facebook.com/pg/100daysintheraw/about/?ref=page_internal
https://www.imdb.com/title/tt3773018/
https://www.youtube.com/watch?v=KEL_iLT4JJI

Dying to Have Known (2006)
Filmmaker Steve Kroschel presents the testimonies of patients, scientists, surgeons and nutritionists who testify to The Gerson Therapy's efficacy in curing cancer and other degenerative diseases. For more information visit:

https://www.facebook.com/DyingToHaveKnown/
https://www.imdb.com/title/tt1782426/
https://www.youtube.com/watch?v=a-JMt9ASvJ4

Eating Like A Nutritarian (2011)
Joel Fuhrman coined the term "Nutritarian" to describe people who eat a diet high in nutrients. In this video he introduces several categories of foods and discusses how to prepare them. For more information visit:

https://www.drfuhrman.com/shop/products/84/eating-like-a-nutritariandvd
https://www.youtube.com/watch?v=UulIQG7SrJE

Fat, Sick & Nearly Dead (2010)
Joe Cross had reached a point in his life where something had to be done. He was obese and was suffering from a chronic autoimmune disease. What do you do when your computer locks up? You reboot it. So, he decided to reboot his life. He documents his 100 pound weight loss and his 60-day juice fast in the documentary film *Fat, Sick & Nearly Dead*. For more information visit:

https://www.fatsickandnearlydead.com/
https://www.facebook.com/FatSickandNearlyDead/
https://www.imdb.com/title/tt1227378/?ref_=nv_sr_1
https://www.rebootwithjoe.com/

Fat, Sick & Nearly Dead 2 (2014)

This one was even more moving and inspiring to me than the first video. Joe meets with experts who present realistic solutions to make long-term sustainable improvements to overall health. For more information visit:

https://www.imdb.com/title/tt3701804/?ref_=tt_rec_tti
http://fatsickandnearlydead2.com/
https://www.rebootwithjoe.com/
https://www.youtube.com/watch?v=UDeTKomY4P8

Food as Medicine (2016)

Food as Medicine is a documentary about the **growing** movement of using food to heal chronic illness. For more information visit:

https://www.imdb.com/title/tt5968588/?ref_=fn_al_tt_1
https://www.youtube.com/watch?v=V80IiKPxxjI
https://www.facebook.com/FoodAsMedicineTheMovie

Food Choices (2016)

In *Food Choices* Michal Siewierski examines how our food choices affect our health and the health of the planet. For more information visit:

https://www.imdb.com/title/tt6039284/?ref_=fn_al_tt_1
https://www.youtube.com/watch?v=9UOw8icI1fY

Food Inc. (2008)

In this documentary Robert Kenner examines America's corporate food industry, and concludes that it produces food that is unhealthy, harmful to the environment, and abusive of both animals and employees. For more information visit:

https://www.imdb.com/title/tt1286537/
http://www.takepart.com/foodinc/index.html
https://www.facebook.com/Foodinc/

Food Matters (2008)

Food Matters examines how food can help or hurt your health. In this documentary, there are several experts (nutritionists, doctors, and journalists) who weigh in on this topic. For more information visit:

https://www.imdb.com/title/tt1528734/
https://www.youtube.com/watch?v=r4DOQ6Xhqss

Forks Over Knives (2011)

This documentary examines the concept that chronic degenerative diseases can be controlled, or even reversed, by adopting a whole-foods, plant-based lifestyle and removing animal-based and processed foods from our diet altogether. For more information visit:

https://www.imdb.com/title/tt1567233/?ref_=fn_al_tt_1
https://www.forksoverknives.com/
https://www.youtube.com/watch?v=O7ijukNzlUg

Heal Your Self: Taking Responsibility for Your Health (2011)
Heal Your Self contains interviews with people who, when faced with serious illness, did just that. They took responsibility for their own health and experienced dramatic healing. For more information visit:

https://www.imdb.com/title/tt2099628/?ref_=fn_al_tt_2
https://www.youtube.com/watch?v=JzgLvy0wrbo
https://www.facebook.com/HealYourSelf.tv

Heal Yourself, Heal the World: The Legacy of Dr. Max Gerson (2013)
John Howard Straus (grandson of Dr. Max Gerson) takes an in-depth look at the Gerson Therapy; how it works and the science behind it. Also included are interviews with several people who have been cured using the therapy. For more information visit:

https://www.youtube.com/watch?v=bI1ZnrPrBW0
https://www.amazon.com/Heal-Yourself-World-Legacy-Gerson/dp/B00JVFRJ9K

Hungry for Change (2012)
Hungry for change exposes the strategies that food manufacturers use to get you hooked on unhealthy junk food. For more information visit:

https://www.imdb.com/title/tt2323551/?ref_=fn_al_tt_1
https://www.youtube.com/watch?v=3MvAM97VDE8
http://www.hungryforchange.tv/

In Defense of Food (2015)
Based on award-winning journalist Michael Pollan's best-selling book, *In Defense of Food* this documentary film explores how the modern diet has been making us sick and what we can do to change it. For more information visit:

https://www.imdb.com/title/tt4785640/plotsummary?ref_=tt_ov_pl
https://www.youtube.com/watch?v=DIW4HJa_gFU

Live Longer, Feel Better (2019)
This is a series of nine videos about the causes and treatments for dementia, depression and diabetes

https://www.livelongerfeelbetter.com/
https://www.facebook.com/LiveLongerFeelBetter/

PlanEAT (2010)
This film discusses the nutritional and environmental benefits of adopting a whole-foods, plant-based diet. It is based on the research of T. Colin Campbell, Caldwell Esselstyn and Gidon Eshel. For more information visit:

https://www.imdb.com/title/tt1467030/?ref_=fn_al_tt_1
https://www.youtube.com/watch?v=qaRhcoEwkDE

Raw Food for Life: Serving Love (2016)

Serving Love shares the stories of people who have experienced profound health benefits by following a raw, plant based lifestyle. For more information visit:

https://www.youtube.com/watch?v=SgNn168duVU
https://www.rawfoodforlife.org/
https://www.veganaustralia.org.au/new_australian_documentary_raw_food_for_life_serving_love

Raw For Life (2007)

Raw For Life is an inspiring documentary that presents the raw food philosophy, the wisdom of eating a raw food diet, and important medical facts regarding eating a raw food diet. For more information visit:

https://www.imdb.com/title/tt1899276/?ref_=fn_al_tt_1
https://www.youtube.com/watch?v=JtvFpF-3B5Q

Simply Raw: Reversing Diabetes in 30 Days (2009)

This documentary film chronicles six people with "incurable" diabetes who were cured using a raw plant-based diet. For more information visit:

https://www.imdb.com/title/tt1587696/
https://www.facebook.com/SimplyRawMovie
https://www.youtube.com/watch?v=P0Le4VjQPlg&fbclid=IwAR3qZjbo7nUYesXYRMggP-lUk7f_9lPw6Os76lqUjIe3-fnjGHEZ3DhlWpk

Super Juice Me! (2014)
What happens when you put 8 people with 22 different health conditions on nothing but freshly extracted juice for 28 Days? They get well! For more information visit:

https://www.youtube.com/watch?v=uwAC6EEx2Y4
https://www.imdb.com/title/tt3529920/

Supersize Me! (2004)
Under a doctor's supervision, Morgan Spurlock personally explores the consequences on his health of a diet consisting solely of McDonald's food for one month. One of his rules was that if he were asked if he wanted to be supersized, he would say yes. For more information visit:

https://www.imdb.com/title/tt0390521/?ref_=nv_sr_1
https://www.youtube.com/watch?v=LOvrkkj_T-I
http://morganspurlock.com/work/super-size-me/

Sustainable (2016)
This documentary film examines America's food and farming system, and talks with an extraordinary farmer who is determined to create a sustainable future. For more information visit:

https://www.imdb.com/title/tt5684868/
https://sustainablefoodfilm.com/

That Sugar Film (2014)

Using himself as the guinea pig, Damon Gameau documents the effects of a high sugar diet on the human body. For more information visit:

https://www.imdb.com/title/tt3892434/?ref_=fn_al_tt_1
https://www.youtube.com/watch?v=vl6JldyduEo

The C Word (2016)

Meghan L. O'Hara follows David Servan-Schreiber M.D. as he applies his anti-cancer principles to his own life and teaches others how to apply them. He was diagnosed with brain cancer and given only two years to live, but he thrived for an additional 20 years by making diet and lifestyle changes. For more information visit:

http://www.thecwordmovie.com/
https://www.youtube.com/watch?v=u4aWw8jCG8I
https://www.imdb.com/title/tt5212792/?ref_=fn_al_tt_3

The Healing Effect (2014)

The Healing Effect is about the healing power of food. The film features interviews with best selling authors and experts who present the simple steps to get you started in changing your life. For more information visit:

https://www.imdb.com/title/tt2629958/?ref_=ttpl_pl_tt
https://www.youtube.com/watch?v=7L_pmVR7ZP8

Vegucated (2011)

Vegucated is a documentary that follows three New Yorkers who agree to adopt a Vegan diet for six weeks in order to learn what it's all about. For more information visit:

https://www.imdb.com/title/tt1814930/
https://www.youtube.com/watch?v=GKzng1_byMY
https://www.getvegucated.com/

What's With Wheat (2018)

This documentary features 15 global experts who shed the light on what is currently happening to our wheat. For more information visit:

https://www.imdb.com/title/tt5882206/
https://www.youtube.com/watch?v=at8iIk14OtM
https://whatswithwheat.com/

A.3 Books

There are hundreds of excellent books available on health and wellness. Here are a few I have found to be valuable resources.

5 Steps to Controlling High Blood Pressure: Your Personal Guide to Preventing and Managing Hypertension, Sheldon G. Sheps, M.D., Mayo Clinic Health Solutions, 2008, Library of Congress Control Number: 2007938953. This book presents a thorough discussion about the causes and treatments for high blood pressure. There are several contributing editors and reviewers for this collaboration.

31-Day Food Revolution: Heal Your Body, Feel Great, and Transform Your World, Ocean Robbins, 2019, ISBN: 978-1-5387-4625-7. Ocean Robbins' plan includes 31 simple and affordable step-by-step actions that provide a road map to healthy, ethical, and sustainable food.

Cholesterol Down: 10 Simple Steps to Lower Your Cholesterol in 4 Weeks Without Prescription Drugs, Janet Bond Brill, Ph.D., R.D., LDN, Three Rivers Press, 2006, ISBN 978-0-307-33911-9. Dr. Brill has been a nutritionists in private practice for many years, specializing in cardiovascular disease prevention. Her ten steps are easy enough for anyone to follow.

Eat to Live: Quick & Easy Cookbook, Joel Furman, M.D., HarperOne, 2017, ISBN 978-0-06-268495-0. This is a beautifully illustrated, full-color cookbook. As the title suggests, Dr. Furman has chosen these recipes because they are quick and easy. Perfect for a guy like me who, at 75 years old, is just learning to cook!

Fat, Sick & Nearly Dead: How Fruits & Vegetables Changed My Life, Joe Cross, Reboot Holdings Pty Ltd., 2011, ISBN 978-1-4507-6478-0. This beautifully illustrated, full-color book is the companion to the *Fat, Sick & Nearly Dead* movie. It provides some interesting background not found in the movie. Foreword by Joel Fuhrman, M.D. and Afterword by Dean Ornish, M.D.

Forks Over Knives: The Cookbook, Del Sroufe, The Experiment, LLC, 2012, ISBN 978-1-61519-061-4. This is the companion cookbook to the documentary *Forks Over Knives*. It has over 300 recipes.

Nutribullet Natural Healing Foods: Supercharge Your Health in Just Seconds a Day! NB-IM011A-18, This is the book that accompanies the Nutribullet blender. It is divided into chapters dealing with the various systems of the body (circulatory system, immune system, digestive system, etc). Each chapter gives helpful background information regarding how the system works, and then provides recipes to boost that specific system.

Prevent and Reverse Heart Disease: The Revolutionary, Scientifically Proven, Nutrition-Based Cure, Caldwell B. Esselstyn, Jr. M.D., Avery, 2008, ISBN 1-58333-272-3. In this book Dr. Esselstyn describes the program he has successfully used to reverse heart disease in several very sick heart patents. This is a nutrition-based program that has a proven success track record. Also, he presents more than 150 great-tasting recipes.

The Complete Book of Juicing: Your Delicious Guide to Youthful Vitality, Michael T. Murray, N.D., Three Rivers Press, 1992, ISBN 0-7615-1126-1. This book provides the background reasoning for eating raw food and juicing. It has chapters on the nutritional properties of fruits and vegetables, juice fasts, how to use juice as medicine, juicing and the immune system, and much more. It also provides fifty juice recipes to get you going on your juicing adventure.

The Complete Idiot's Guide to Eating Raw: A Fresh Approach to Eating Well with Over 150 Delicious Recipes, Mark Reinfeld, Bo Rinaldi, and Jennifer Murray, Alpha Books, 2008, ISBN 978-1-59257-771-2. This book explains the benefits of raw foods over cooked foods and has over 150 recipes. It also describes the techniques involved in raw food preparation.

The Engine 2 Diet: The Texas Firefighter's 28-Day Save-Your-Life Plan that Lowers Cholesterol and Burns Away the Pounds, Rip Esselstyn, Grand Central Life & Style, 2009, ISBN 978-0-446-50669-4. This excellent book is instructive and motivating. The first two parts explain the program with plenty of tips to help you succeed, and the third part consists of recipes and meal plans.

The Vegan Starter Kit: Everything You Need To Know About Plant-Based Eating, Neal D. Barnard, MD, FACC, 2018, ISBN 978-1-5387-4740-7. The Vegan Starter Kit is a practical guide that makes plant-based eating easy and fun.

To Your Health: A Guide to Heart-Smart Living, American Heart Association, Clarkston Potter Publishers, 2001, ISBN 0-609-80702-1. This practical little book was given to me while I was in the hospital recovering from triple-bypass open-heart surgery. It is loaded with realistic, helpful information, and was a great help to me as I started my recovery.

Appendix B: Answers to the Ingredients Quiz

1. Signature Care: Antacid Plus Gas Relief
2. Ramen Noodle Soup (Chicken Flavor)
3. Morning Star Farms Veggie Berger
4. Apple
5. Safeway Signature Select Pizza
6. Aveeno Active Naturals Body Wash, Fragrance Free, Dermatologist Recommended
7. Banana
8. Idahoan Baby Reds Mashed Potatoes
9. Organics Popping Corn

Appendix C: Understanding Blood Pressure

A blood pressure measurement consists of two numbers:

1. The higher number (systolic) represents the pressure when he heart contracts.
2. The lower number (diastolic) represents the pressure when the heart relaxes between beats.

The numbers represented millimeters of mercury (mm Hg).

Table C-1 shows how various blood pressure levels are categorized. If you search the Internet, you will find that different organizations categorize these levels somewhat differently. I took the numbers for Table C-1 from the American Heart Association's book *To Your Health: A Guide to Heart-Smart Living* (2001). My primary care physician is happy when my systolic pressure is under 140.

Systolic (mm Hg)	Diastolic (mm Hg)	Category
Less than 120	Less than 80	Ideal
120 - 129	80 - 85	Normal
130 - 139	85 - 89	Prehypertension
140 - 159	90 - 99	Stage 1 Hypertension
160 - 179	100 - 109	Stage 2 Hypertension
180 or higher	110 or higher	Hypertensive Crisis

Table A-1 Blood Pressure Categories

Keeping your blood pressure in the normal range is very important. If your blood pressure is too high you are at risk for stroke, kidney failure and heart failure.

Appendix D: Body Mass Index and Body Fat Percentage

Everyone is unique in terms of musculature, bone size, gender and age, but there is a simple rule of thumb regarding healthy weight for any individual. It's called "Body Mass Index."

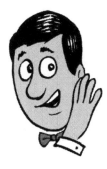

"In my opinion there is a big difference between the arbitrary BMI number and a person's actual health based on body composition and other factors, but it is a good starting point and a quick rule of thumb."

D.1 Body Mass Index (BMI)

The body mass index relates a persons weight and height. It is determined by dividing weight by the square of height. This results in the following formulas for pounds or kilograms.

When using pounds and inches, we need to use a correction factor of 703. So here are the formulas.

1. Using pounds and inches: [weight (lb) / (height in inches)^2] x 703
2. Using kilograms and meters: weight (kg) / (height in meters)^2

For example: A person who is 5' 4" and weighs 140 pounds:

BMI = (140 / 64²) x 703
BMI = 24

Table D-1 summarizes the BMI categories.

BMI	CATEGORY
Less than 18.5	Underweight
18.5 - 25	Normal weight
25 - 30	Overweight
30 - 40	Obese
40 or greater	Morbidly Obese

Table D-1 BMI Categories

If you don't like doing math, you can use Table D-2 or D-3 to find your BMI.

Height (in)	Weight (lb)								
58	91	96	100	105	110	115	119	124	129
59	94	99	104	109	114	119	124	128	133
60	97	102	107	112	118	123	128	133	138
61	100	106	111	116	122	127	132	137	143
62	104	109	115	120	126	131	136	142	147
63	107	113	118	124	130	135	141	146	152
64	110	116	122	128	134	140	145	151	157
65	114	120	126	132	138	144	150	156	162
66	118	124	130	136	142	148	155	161	167
67	121	127	134	140	146	153	159	166	172
68	125	131	138	144	151	158	164	171	177
69	128	135	142	149	155	162	169	176	182
70	132	139	146	153	160	167	174	181	188
71	136	143	150	157	165	172	179	186	193
72	140	147	154	162	169	177	184	191	199
73	144	151	159	166	174	182	189	197	204
74	148	155	163	171	179	186	194	202	210
75	152	160	168	176	184	192	200	208	216
76	156	164	172	180	189	197	205	213	221
BMI	**19**	**20**	**21**	**22**	**23**	**24**	**25**	**26**	**27**
	Normal Weight						Overweight		

Table D-2 BMI Chart

Height (in)	Weight (lb)								
58	134	138	143	148	153	158	162	167	172
59	138	143	148	153	158	163	168	173	178
60	143	148	153	158	163	168	174	179	184
61	148	153	158	164	169	174	180	185	190
62	153	158	164	169	175	180	186	191	196
63	158	163	169	175	180	186	191	197	202
64	163	169	174	180	186	192	197	204	209
65	168	174	180	186	192	198	204	210	215
66	173	179	186	192	198	204	210	216	222
67	178	185	191	198	204	211	217	223	228
68	184	190	197	203	210	216	223	230	235
69	189	196	203	209	216	223	230	236	242
70	195	202	209	216	222	229	236	243	248
71	200	208	215	222	229	236	243	250	255
72	206	213	221	228	235	242	250	258	263
73	212	219	227	235	242	250	257	265	270
74	218	225	233	241	249	256	264	272	277
75	224	232	240	248	256	264	272	279	284
76	230	238	246	254	263	271	279	287	292
BMI	28	29	30	31	32	33	34	35	36
	Overweight		Obese						

Table D-3 BMI Chart (cont.)

D.2 Body Fat Percentage

BMI is a handy measurement, but it doesn't take into account body composition - especially body fat percentage. Figure D-1 shows the fancy scale that I purchased called "Body

Composition Monitor." It is a BIA machine (see definition below) that measures or computes the following:

1. Body fat percentage
2. Body water percentage
3. Viscera fat
4. Bone mass
5. Muscle mass
6. Physique rating
7. Metabolic age

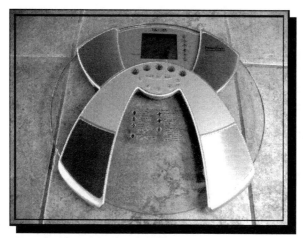

Figure D-1 Body Composition Monitor

D.2.1 Determining Body Fat Percentage

Body fat can be measured in several different ways. The four most common methods are:

1. **Hydrodensitometry** is based on weighing a person in air and then again while immersed in water. These two values together with the amount of water displaced can be used to determine the person's specific gravity and percent body fat.

2. **Calipers** measure skin fold thickness to determine the amount of fat under the skin.
3. **DEXA** (dual energy x-ray absorptiometry) uses low-dose x-rays to measure bone and soft tissue mass. This is the "gold standard" but it requires expensive equipment and a trained technician to interpret the results.
4. **BIA** (bioelectrical impedance analysis) passes a low level current through the body. The signal passes much faster through lean muscle than fat because muscle contains 70-75% of the body's water and fat contains almost no water. This is the simple and inexpensive circuit that is built into my scales.

D.2.2 Body Fat Percentage Ranges

A certain amount of body fat is essential for health. It cushions the joints, protects internal organs, helps regulate body temperature, is involved in the manufacture of hormones, and acts as an energy reserve. The only problem today in America is that, because of our lifestyle and food choices, we are storing too much fat!

Table D-4 summarize body fat categories for men and women. These categories vary somewhat by age, and different sources will cite different numbers, but these are fairly good rules of thumb.

Men (% fat)	Women (% fat)	Category
2-4%	10-12%	Essential Fat
6-13%	13-20%	Athletes
14-17%	21-24%	Healthy
18-25%	25-31%	Acceptable
26+%	32+%	Obese

Table D-4 Body Fat Percentage Categories

Appendix E: Understanding Your Blood Test Results

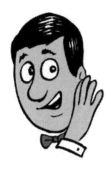

"As I mentioned in the Preface, I am not a medical doctor, and I wouldn't presume to give medical advice. But since I started taking responsibility for my own health, I wanted to know a little more about all those mysterious numbers you see in the lab printout. I'll share with you what I have learned that may help eliminate some of the mystery."

A whole book could be written about interpreting blood test results (in fact several have been). I'll share with you just a few of the most important numbers. Consider this as just a brief overview. You can always dive deeper with Internet searches or by talking with your doctor.

The human body has such an amazingly complex set of biological and chemical interactions. It just blows me away! Some of the substances that are measured in the blood are also measured in the urine (Appendix F). So, bottom line, everything is interconnected. I have always loved mathematics, engineering, and astronomy, but I'm finding out that the human body is as complex (and as interesting) as any of the physical sciences.

I used to think that lab results were too confusing and impossible for the average Joe Blow like me to understand, so I would just leave it up to my doctor to interpret them for me. The actual numbers were a complete mystery to me. All I knew was that my doctor said they were either good or bad. But now that I have taken responsibility for my own health, I am interested in knowing (at least a little bit) what all these numbers mean. This will be a high-level overview.

The lab numbers give a good snapshot of what's going on with your major organs and systems including: liver, kidneys, bone marrow, thyroid gland, parathyroid glands, pancreas, arteries and immune system. If all of these organs and systems are functioning properly it is likely that you are in good health.

If one or more of the numbers is significantly out of the "normal" range there is a reason for it, and your doctor will want to investigate it further. He may recommend some drugs to bring the number back in line.

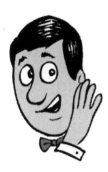

"To me, that's just treating the symptom instead of determining what is causing that abnormal reading and treating the cause, but I recognize that there are times when the symptom needs to be treated - like with dangerously high blood pressure."

Each of us is unique, and therefore there is a range of values for each of these measurements, not just a single number that you should strive for. In fact the upper and lower limits for normal values are "soft" numbers. If you are slightly outside that range, your doctor will probably not be overly concerned.

For each of the tests:
1. Result = the actual reading. There will be a "High" or "Low" notation if the results are out of the normal range.
2. Reference Range = the range of values considered to be normal.
3. Units = the units in which the reading is expressed.

Table E-1 summarizes the abbreviations used for the units, and Table E-2 defines the prefixes for the various powers of ten.

Units	Meaning
%	percentage
mg/g	milligrams per gram
mg/dL	milligrams per deciliter (1/10th liter)
mEq/L	milliequivalents per liter
mmoL/L	millimoles per liter
umol/L	micromoles per Liter
g/dL	grams per deciliter (1/10th liter)
U/L	units per liter
mL/min	milliliters per minute
ng/mL	nanograms per milliliter
EU/dl	equivalent units per deciliter (1/10th liter)
/HPF	high-power field
/LPF	low-power field
K/cmm or K/mm^3	Thousand per cubic millimeter
M/cmm or M/mm^3	Million per cubic millimeter
fL	Femtoliters or 10^{-15} liters
pg	picograms (10^{-12} grams)
uU/mL	microunits per milliliter

Table E-1 Abbreviations for the Units

Prefix	Power of Ten
giga	10^9
mega	10^6
kilo	10^3
milli	10^{-3}
micro	10^{-6}
nano	10^{-9}
pico	10^{-12}
femto	10^{-15}

Table E-2 Prefixes for the Powers of Ten

Some of this stuff may seem pretty technical at first. That's why I stuck in an appendix. I have tried to make it as easy and painless as possible. Just take it a little at a time. If you are serious about taking responsibility for your own health, you will probably be curious about what all these strange numbers mean.

E.1 Complete Blood Count (CBC)

The Complete Blood Count (CBC) includes parameters for red blood cells (RBC), white blood cells (WBC), and platelets. It is a measure of the health of your bone morrow and immune system.

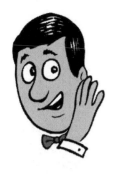

"Believe it or not, your bones have lots of blood vessels in them. That's how the blood gets from the bone marrow into the blood stream. So, your bones are not just a hard chalky stick."

E.1.1 Red Blood Cells

Red blood cells are filled with hemoglobin and carry oxygen to the cells. Anemia is a condition in which the number of red blood cells or the amount of hemoglobin in them is low; therefore the blood can't supply the cells with adequate amounts of oxygen.

E.1.2 Red Blood Cell Count

There should be between 4.7 million and 6.1 million red blood cells per cubic millimeter of blood. If there aren't enough red blood cells, a person will become anemic.

Test Name: RBC
Result: 5.78
Units: M/cmm
Reference Range: (4.70-6.10)

E.1.3 Hemoglobin

Hemoglobin is an iron containing protein in the red blood cells that carries oxygen from the lungs to the tissues.

Test Name: HGB
Result: 19.5 High

Units: g/dL
Reference Range: (14.0-18.0)

E.1.4 Hematocrit

Blood is composed of red blood cells and white blood cells suspended in a clear fluid called serum. The hematocrit test (HCT) determines what percentage of the blood is composed of red blood cells. Too low indicates anemia, and too high indicates a rare form of blood cancer called Polycythemia Vera.

Test Name: HCT
Result: 56.9 High
Units: %
Reference Range: (42.0-52.0)

E.1.5 Mean Corpuscular Volume (RBC Size)

You may have enough red blood cells, but are they healthy?

There are conditions that cause the red blood cells to be too big or too small. If you have an iron deficiency, the red blood cells will be too small. If you don't have enough vitamin B-12, your red blood cells will be too large.

Test Name: MCV
Result: 98.4
Units: fL
Reference Range: (80-100)

E.1.6 Mean Corpuscular Hemoglobin Concentration

This measurement tells how much hemoglobin is in each red blood cell.

Test Name: MCH
Result: 33.8
Units: pg
Reference Range: (26-34)

E.1.7 Red Cell Distribution Width (RDW)

RDW tell about the roundness and regularity of the red blood cells. If all the red blood cells are about the same size the "distribution" is very small. If there are many different sizes of red blood cells the distribution will be wide. In people with sickle cell anemia the cells are not round.

Test Name: RDW
Result: 12.7
Units: %
Reference Range: (11-15)

E.1.8 Platelet Count

Platelets are made in the bone marrow. They are the cells responsible for clotting your blood. With infections or bleeding disorders the platelet count goes down. When the platelet count gets below 50,000 people will bleed and bruise more easily.

Test Name: PLATELET
Result: 202
Units: K/cmm

Reference Range: (150-440)

E.1.9 Mean Platelet Volume

Large platelets are often the sign of a bleeding disorder.

Test Name: MPV
Result: 9.1
Units: fL
Reference Range: (7.4-10.4)

E.1.10 White Blood Cells and the Immune System

White blood cells fight infections. Your white blood cell count will increase if you have an infection or a severe inflammatory reaction.

There are five different types of white blood cells, and each type has a specific function.

1. Neutrophils: Neutrophils are the most numerous of the white blood cells. They make up about 56 percent of all white blood cells. They eat bacteria.

2. Lymphocytes: Lymphocytes play a major roll in the antibody production of the immune system. They typically reside in the lymphatic system. They defend you against viral infections.

3. Monocytes: Monocytes are the largest type of white blood cell. Because of their large size they can digest large foreign particles including dead cells.

4. Eosinophils: Eosinophils release toxins that kill pathogens like parasites and worms. High Eosinophils levels are associated with allergic reactions.

5. Basophils: Basophils release histamines that dilate the blood vessels allowing more immune cells to reach the area of injury.

E.1.11 White Blood Cell Count (WBC)

WBC refers to the total number of white blood cells. This includes all five types. The normal range is from 4.0-11.0 K/mm^3. If a person has appendicitis, the white blood cell count could spike up to 15,000 cells per cubic millimeter of blood.

Test Name: WBC
Result: 7.9
Units: K/cmm
Reference Range: (4.0-11.0)

E.1.12 Neutrophil Count and % (Bacterial Infections)

If you have a bacterial infection like pneumonia, tonsillitis, or appendicitis, your neutrophil count will spike. So, a high neutrophil count indicates an infection in the body. These little guys are out there trying to eat up the bacteria.

Test Name: NEUT #
Result: 5.8
Units: K/cmm
Reference Range: (2.0-7.0)

Test Name: NEUT %

Result: 73.6 High
Units: %
Reference Range: (40.0-70.0)

E.1.13 Lymphocyte Count and % (Viral Infections)

Lymphocytes are small cells with a large nucleus. They go after viruses. If you have a viral infection like the mumps, measles, or chickenpox, your lymphocyte count will spike.

Test Name: LYMPH #
Result: 1.2
Units: K/cmm
Reference Range: (1.0-3.0)

Test Name: LYMPH %
Result: 15.0 Low
Units: %
Reference Range: (20.0-40.0)

E.1.14 Monocyte Count and %

Monocytes support a healthy immune system by ingesting and destroying pathogens. An abnormally high monocytes reading is called monocytosis. High monocyte levels indicate an infection in the body such as tuberculosis or Epstein Bar virus (mononucleosis). It can also be a sign of inflammatory bowel disease and certain types of cancer.

Test Name: MONO #
Result: 0.7
Units: K/cmm
Reference Range: (0.2-1.0)

Test Name: MONO %
Result: 8.6
Units: %
Reference Range: (2.0-10.0)

E.1.15 Eosinophil Count and % (Parasites and Allergies)

If you visit a country known to have contaminated water and come back with an elevated eosinophil count, it's likely you picked up a parasite.

Test Name: EOS #
Result: 0.2
Units: K/cmm
Reference Range: (<0.7)

Test Name: EOS %
Result: 2.3
Units: %
Reference Range: (<5.0)

E.1.16 Basophile Count and % (Allergic Reactions)

Basophiles contain an intense blue pigment. A high basophile count is an indicator of allergic reaction, inflammation, or cancer.

Test Name: BASO #
Result: 0.0
Units: K/cmm
Reference Range: (<0.2)

Test Name: BASO %
Result: 0.5
Units: %
Reference Range: (<2.0)

E.2 Comprehensive Metabolic Profile (CMP)

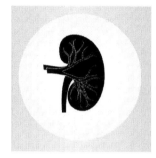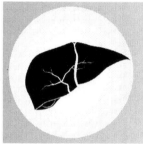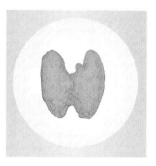

The comprehensive metabolic profile (blood chemistry) gives important information about the chemical makeup of your blood, and it reveals the health of three major organs: the kidneys, liver, and parathyroid.

Sections E.2.1 - E.2.7 relate to kidney (renal) function. The kidneys maintain mineral balance in the blood stream.

Section E.2.8 relates to parathyroid function. The parathyroid regulates calcium levels in the blood,

Sections E.2.9 - E.2.14 relate to liver function. The liver is often called the "Master Chemist" because it performs thousands of chemical reactions. The liver makes proteins like albumin, and it gets rid of wastes like bilirubin.

E.2.1 Sodium (Kidneys)

The numbers for sodium reflects the water balance in your body. If you are dehydrated your sodium value will go up. If you are drinking too much water you will dilute out the sodium and your sodium values will go down.

Test Name: SODIUM
Result: 138
Units: mEq/L
Reference Range: (137-145)

E.2.2 Potassium (Kidneys)

Potassium is an electrolyte that helps control muscle and nerve activity, and maintain fluid levels. Potassium is found in many foods, such as bananas, apricots, and avocados, and is part of a healthy diet. But eating excessive amounts of potassium-rich foods can lead to health problems.

Too much potassium in the blood, a condition known as hyperkalemia, may indicate:

1. Kidney disease
2. Burns or other traumatic injuries
3. Addison's disease
4. Type 1 diabetes
5. The effect of medicines, such as diuretics or antibiotics

Too little potassium in the blood, a condition known as hypokalemia, may indicate:

1. A diet too low in potassium
2. Alcoholism
3. Loss of bodily fluids from diarrhea, vomiting, or use of diuretics
4. Aldosteronism, a hormonal disorder that causes high blood pressure

Test Name: POTASSIUM
Result: 4.4
Units: mEq/L
Reference Range: (3.5-5.1)

E.2.3 Chloride (Kidneys)

Chloride values can vary quite a bit as the kidneys do their job. You can pretty much disregard the chloride numbers.

Test Name: CHLORIDE
Result: 102
Units: mEq/L
Reference Range: (98-108)

E.2.4 Carbon Dioxide (Kidneys)

Carbon dioxide values can vary quite a bit as the kidneys do their job. You can pretty much disregard the carbon dioxide numbers.

Test Name: CARBON DIOXIDE

Result: 28
Units: mmoL/L
Reference Range: (22-30)

E.2.5 Blood Urea Nitrogen (Kidneys)

This is an important number. Blood urea nitrogen (B.U.N.) is a waste product from protein metabolism. It's the ammonia from amino acids. When we burn protein for energy, the byproduct is ammonia (a very toxic compound). So your kidneys take that ammonia and combine it with carbon dioxide to form urea, which is much less toxic to your body. If your kidneys are healthy, your B.U.N. readings will fall in the normal range. Actually, the lower the better.

When people go into kidney failure the B.U.N. goes up. In a dialysis unit where people have no kidney function you will see B.U.N. numbers of 100 or 120.

Test Name: UREA NITROGEN (B.U.N.)
Result: 11
Units: mg/dL
Reference Range: (7-20)

E.2.6 Creatinine (Kidneys)

This is an important number. Creatinine is a waste product from the muscles. Every time you move a muscle a little bit of creatinine enters the blood stream, and your kidneys get rid of it. Healthy kidneys keep the creatinine well below 1.25. If both the B.U.N. and creatinine numbers are high, it's likely that the person is in kidney failure.

Test Name: CREATININE
Result: 0.96
Units: mg/dL
Reference Range: (0.52-1.25)

You should typically see a ratio of B.U.N. to creatinine of 10 - 20.

E.2.7 ESTIMATED GFR (eGFR) (Kidneys)

The estimated glomerular filtration rate (eGFR) tells us how many milliliters of blood the kidneys filter each minute. This is an "estimated value" because it is not measured directly; it is computed using a complex formula. If this number is greater than 60, that's a good indication that all of the other kidney numbers are reliable.

We like to see the eGFR greater than 60 mL/min. If it is lower than that we are looking at kidney disease. This is serious! Table 2-2 summarizes the eGFR values and how they relate to kidney disease.

eGFR Value	Kidney Disease
>60 mL/min	Normal kidney function
60 - 30 mL/min	Mild renal disease (Stage III)
30 - 15 mL/min	Moderate renal disease (Stage IV)
<15 mL/min	Severe renal disease (Stage V)

Table E 2-2 eGFR Values and Kidney Disease

Test Name: EGFR
Result: >60

Units: mL/min
Reference Range: (>60)

E.2.8 Calcium (Parathyroid)

On the backside of your thyroid are four little glands called parathyroid glands. Calcium levels in the blood are determined by your parathyroid glands. It does NOT reflect the health of your bones. Calcium plays many important roles in the body including blood clotting, muscle contraction, and heart function. Because calcium is critical to these important functions, your body maintains calcium levels pretty strictly. If there is too much calcium in the blood the excess will be stored in your bones. If there is too little calcium your body will draw it from your bones. So, your bones act like a savings and loan for calcium.

Test Name: CALCIUM
Result: 9.4
Units: mg/dL
Reference Range: (8.4-10.2)

E.2.9 Total Protein (Liver)

The total protein in the blood is made up of two proteins, albumin and globulin.

Test Name: TOTAL PROTEIN
Result: 7.0
Units: g/dL
Reference Range: (6.3-8.2)

E.2.10 Albumin (Liver)

Albumin keeps the osmotic forces in the blood constant. When people are alcoholic, in liver failure, or have liver cancer they loose the ability to synthesize albumin and levels drop below 3.3 g/dL. A healthy liver will produce an abundant amount of albumin.

Test Name: ALBUMIN
Result: 4.3
Units: g/dL
Reference Range: (3.5-5.0)

E.2.11 Globulin (Liver)

Globulin is the other protein in the blood. Elevated globulin levels are a sign of cancer, infection, or other serious conditions.

Test Name: GLOBULIN
Result: 2.7
Units: g/dL
Reference Range: (2.0-3.0)

E.2.12 Albumin/Globulin Ratio (Liver)

With liver disease the albumin goes down and the globulin goes up, so the ratio gets quite small. This ratio tells us how well the liver is synthesizing these two proteins.

Test Name: ALBUMIN/GLOBULIN RATIO
Result: 1.6
Units: %
Reference Range: (1.0-2.2)

E.2.13 Bilirubin Total (Liver)

Bilirubin is a yellow pigment waste product that the liver gets rid of. If the liver is sick and can't get rid of the bilirubin it leaks into the tissues and the person turns yellow. That's called jaundice. If the total bilirubin is > 3.0 mg/dL, the laboratory will automatically perform a direct bilirubin test.

Test Name: BILIRUBIN, TOTAL
Result: 1.5 High
Units: mg/dL
Reference Range: (0.2-1.3)

E.2.14 AST (SGOT) and ALT (SGPT) (Liver)

These are liver cell enzymes. They belong in the liver, not out in the blood stream. When the liver is inflamed for any reason (hepatitis, alcohol, Tylenol, statin drugs, seatbelt injury) these enzymes will spill out into the blood stream.

Test Name: AST (SGOT)
Result: 22
Units: U/L
Reference Range: (0-40)

Test Name: ALT (SGPT)
Result: 14
Units: U/L
Reference Range: (0-50)

E.3 Thyroid Profile

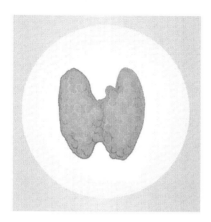

The thyroid regulates your metabolism by secreting thyroxin. This hormone determines the rate that cells burn energy (glucose). Having either too fast or too slow of a metabolism is not good.

If you have too much thyroxin (hyperthyroidism) you will have a fast heart rate, a fever and a flushed face. Uncontrolled, it can lead to heart failure.

If you have too little thyroxin (hypothyroidism) you will have a slow heart rate, be cold, retain fluid, and be lethargic. This can lead to a different type of heart failure.

E.3.1 Thyroid Stimulating Hormone (TSH)

How does the thyroid know how much thyroxin to put out? At the base of your brain is a gland called the "pituitary" that senses the thyroxin level in the blood. If the level is too low it will excrete thyroid stimulating hormone (TSH) telling the thyroid to release more thyroxin. When the level is high enough it will stop secreting TSH.

The thyroid makes and stores T4. This is not the active form of thyroxin; it is stored in the thyroid waiting to be released. When it is released into the blood stream the liver and kidneys will convert it to T3, which is the active form of thyroxin that stimulated the cells to burn sugar. Sometimes T3 and T4 levels are measured, but if you had only one test performed it would be for TSH.

Test Name: TSH
Result: 1.7
Units: uU/mL
Reference Range: (1.3-4.2)

E.4 Pancreas Function

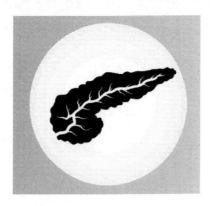

E.4.1 Blood Sugar Level (Glucose)

The pancreas puts out insulin to keep your blood sugar normal. If you were fasting the previous evening you should wake up with a blood sugar below 100. High blood sugar levels are an indicator of diabetes.

Test Name: GLUCOSE
Result: 109 High
Units: mg/dL
Reference Range: (74-106)

E.4.2 Hemoglobin A1C

The glucose test is just a snapshot in time, but the hemoglobin A1C test tells your average blood sugar level (glucose level) over the past two to three months. How can you tell the average level over the past three months from only one reading? The average red cell lifetime is three months, so at any given time some of your red blood cells are very young, and some are three months old. The A1C test tells you the percentage of the hemoglobin in your blood stream that is sticky with sugar.

The American Diabetes Association goal is <7%. If your A1C is higher than 7% you have diabetes.

Test Name: HEMOGLOBIN A1C
Result: 5.8
Units: %
Reference Range: (4.0-6.0)

E.5 Lipids

Cholesterol has a bad reputation, but it is an essential building block in the human body. Your liver produces cholesterol, and your body uses it to build important substances, including hormones. The problem arises when it becomes oxidized (like with smoking) and starts to stick to the artery walls.

E.5.1 Total Cholesterol

Total cholesterol is made up of LDL cholesterol, HDL cholesterol, and triglycerides.

Test Name: TOTAL CHOLESTEROL
Result: 205 High
Units: mg/dL
Reference Range: (<200)

Total Cholesterol (mg/dL)
    Desirable < 200
    Borderline 200 – 239
    High >240

E.5.2 Triglycerides

Test Name: TRIGLYCERIDE
Result: 138
Units: mg/dL
Reference Range: (<150)

Triglycerides (mg/dL)
    Desirable < 150
    Borderline High 150 – 199
    High 200 – 499
    Very High > 500

E.5.3 HDL

High Density Lipoproteins (HDL) is the "good" cholesterol. You want this as high as possible. It is protective because it pulls the plaque out of the arteries.

It's interesting to note that for a healthy Vegan to have low HDL is not a bad thing. Why not? Because they don't have a lot of plaque in their arteries that needs to be removed, so their HDL is low. So, the question is not "How high is your cholesterol?" The question is "How clean are your arteries?" Have your doctor look at your retina. The back of the eye is the only place where you can look at blood vessels directly. If there is plaque building up, he will see it. If you have plaques in your retina, you probably have plaques everywhere!

Another good test for plaque buildup is to get an ultrasound of the carotid artery in your neck and the abdominal aorta.

Test Name: DIRECT HDL
Result: 39
Units: mg/dL
Reference Range: (30-60)

HDL (mg/dL)
Desirable > 40
Considered to offer some protection > 60

Considered to be a significant independent risk factor < 35

E.5.4 LDL

Low Density Lipoproteins (LDL) is the "bad" cholesterol. You want them as low as possible because they contribute to plaque buildup in the arteries.

LDL (mg/dL)
Desirable < 100
Desirable for heart patients < 70

E.5.5 Calculating LDL Cholesterol

If you purchase a home cholesterol test kit it will probably give you readings for total cholesterol, HDL and triglycerides but not for LDL. With the following simple formula you can calculate your LDL cholesterol.

LDL = Total Cholesterol – HDL – 1/5 Triglycerides

For example if your Total Cholesterol = 150, HDL = 42, and Triglycerides = 120 then:

LDL = 150 – 42 – (1/5 x 120)
    = 150 – 42 – 24
    = 84

E.6 Other Blood Markers

E.6.1 Vitamin B-12 and Homocysteine

Homocysteine is the waste product of amino acid metabolism that builds up in the blood stream. If it builds up too high it can damage your arteries.

Vitamin B-12 and homocysteine are usually measured together because the B-12 numbers are often incorrect for people taking blue-green algae or sea vegetables. These plants contain vitamin B-12 "analogues" (not actually B-12) that can fool the test.

Vitamin B-12 is used in the metabolism of homocysteine. Adequate amounts of B-12 will help to keep the homocysteine level low. Therefore, the homocystein level tells us how well the active vitamin B-12 is functioning. If a person has high homocystein levels, they are deficient in vitamin B-12. Conversely, if your homocystein level is nice and low, you have plenty of vitamin B-12. If you are a vegetarian you should supplement B-12 because plants don't produce it.

Test Name: VITAMIN B-12
Result: 618
Units: pg/mL
Reference Range: (165-912)

Test Name: HOMOCYSTEINE
Result: 10.8
Units: umol/L
Reference Range: (5.0-13.0)

E.6.2 Vitamin D

Vitamin D is critical for healthy bones, but it's also involved in hundreds of important reactions throughout the body including: stabilizing membranes, helping to prevent cancer, helping to slow the progression of Alzheimer's disease, and boosting immune function. As with B-12, if you are a vegetarian you should supplement with vitamin D. It's also a good idea to spent some time out in the sun.

Test Name: VITAMIN D 25-HYDROXY
Result: 45
Units: ng/mL
Reference Range: (30-70)

E.6.3 Prostate Specific Antigen (PSA)

This test is a screening tool for prostate cancer, but there is some controversy regarding this test. Many prestigious medical organizations support PSA screening (American Urological Association and American Cancer Society), and many are against it (National Cancer Institute and Center for Disease Control and Prevention).

Men with prostate cancer may have up to ten times the amount of this protein than men without cancer, but several non-cancer conditions (such as an enlarged or inflamed prostate) can produce a high reading. This can result in unnecessary biopsy or unnecessary cancer treatment. So, the PSA test alone is not used to diagnose prostate cancer. It needs to be used in conjunction with other test such as a digital rectal exam (the dreaded rubber glove test) and biopsy.

Some symptoms should not be ignored such as trouble urinating or blood in the urine.

The normal range is 0 to 4 ng/mL, but more important than a single reading is to understand what the PSA is doing over time.

Test Name: PROSTATIC SPECIFIC ANTIGEN
Result: 2.6
Units: ng/mL
Reference Range: (<4.0)

E.6.4 Uric Acid and LDH

These are substances that spill out into the blood stream when tissue is being destroyed. It could be from a cancer or from an infection that is abscessed. If your numbers are in the normal range they are from natural cell "turnover." Uric acid buildup can result in painful crystals in the joints called gout.

Test Name: URIC ACID
Result: 6.0
Units: ug/dL
Reference Range: (2.6-8.0)

Test Name: LDH (Lactic Acid Dehydrogenase)
Result: 195

Units: U/L
Reference Range: (140-230)

E.6.5 Inflammation CRP and Sedimentation Rate

C-Reactive Protein in the blood is a sign of inflammation. Readings should be less than 5 ng/L.

Test Name: CRP C-Reactive Protein
Result: 2.5
Units: ng/L
Reference Range: <5

To determine the sedimentation rate, a blood sample is mixed with an anticoagulant to keep it from clotting and the mixture is drawn up into a calibrated tube. The plasma rises to the top and the red blood cells settle to the bottom. The sedimentation rate is how quickly the red blood cells settle out of the solution. Normally blood is thick and the red blood cells should not fall quickly. The "sed rate" is how far they fall (how many millimeters in the calibrated tube) in an hour. An elevated "sed rate" is a sign of inflammation.

Test Name: Sedimentation Rate
Result: 15
Units: mm/Hr
Reference Range: < 20 mm/Hr for a male and < 30 mm/Hr for a female

E.6.6 MCHC

The mean corpuscular hemoglobin concentration (MCHC) is the average concentration of hemoglobin in your red blood cells.

Hemoglobin is the protein that allows red blood cells to carry oxygen to tissues within your body. This test is done to help diagnose anemia.

Test Name: MCHC
Result: 34.3
Units: g/dL
Reference Range: (33-37)

Appendix F: Interpreting Urinalysis

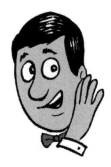

"As with your blood test results, urinalysis numbers can be a little confusing, but let's try and make some sense out of them."

Urinalysis (UA) is the contraction of the terms "urine" and "analysis." It is the physical, chemical, and microscopic analysis of a urine sample. It can be used to evaluate several different medical problems including:

1. Kidney failure
2. Urinary tract infections (UTIs)
3. Kidney and ureteral stones
4. GU malignancy
5. Acid-based disorders
6. Abnormalities of volume status
7. Rhabdomyolysis
8. Response to alkalization therapy

UA results can be divided into three broad categories;

1. Gross Inspection
2. Dipstick
3. Microscopy

F.1 Gross Inspection

Gross inspection includes color and turbidity (how clear the urine is).

F.1.1 Color

Your urine will change color under different circumstances. If you are well hydrated it will be a light color, but if you are dehydrated it will be darker. That's why it will typically be darker first thing in the morning. Also, urine color can be influenced by several other factors including medical conditions, medications, and even foods. Table F-1 summarizes potential causes for different colors of urine.

Color	Potential Causes
Red	Medical Conditions: bleeding, porphyria, factitious disorder Meds: rifampin, phenytoin, phenazopyridine Foods: beets
Orange	Medical Conditions: hyperbilirubinemia Meds: rifampin Foods: excessive vitamin A or vitamin B complex
Brown or Black	Medical Conditions: Any condition causing red or orange urine if severe enough Meds: metronidazole, nitrofurantpin, senna, sorbitol
Green	Medical Conditions: Urinary tract infections (UTIs) Meds: methylene blue, propofol, amitriptyline, promethazine, metoclopramide, indomethacin Foods: asparagus, blue food dyes (blue mixed with yellow results in green)

Table F-1 Potential Causes for Various Colors in the Urine

Test Name: URINE COLOR
Result: YELLOW

F.1.2 Turbidity

Turbidity means how clear or cloudy the urine looks. Turbid urine may indicate: urinary tract infection (UTI) or precipitated crystals.

Test Name: APPEARANCE
Result: CLEAR
Units: --

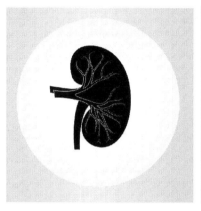 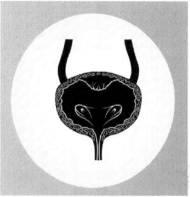

The dipstick is a reagent strip that is dipped into the urine. This will trigger a series of color changes along its length that indicate the presence and concentration of various substances in the urine. Specific properties tested for include:

1. Specific gravity
2. pH
3. Glucose
4. Heme
5. Protein
6. Leukocyte
7. Nitrites
8. Ketones and
9. Bilirubin

Specific gravity is a measure of density. It is the density of urine divided by the density of water as follows:

$$\text{Specific Gravity} = \text{Density of urine/Density of water}$$

Urine is mostly composed of water, but it does contain a few other compounds like electrolytes and urea that make it slightly denser than water. Significant amounts of protein or glucose in the urine will increase its density.

If the urine has a specific gravity close to 1.001 it is very dilute. This condition can be caused by excessive hydration, diabetes, or ATN where the kidneys have lost the ability to concentrate urine.

A specific gravity of 1.035 implies the opposite. This condition can be caused by dehydration, SIADH (syndrome of inappropriate anti-diuretic hormone), CHF, cirrhosis, too much glucose (glycosuria), or too much protein in the urine (proteinuria), or recent administration of IV contrast.

A specific gravity that is consistently around 1.010 is an indication of kidney failure.

Test Name: SPECIFIC GRAVITY
Result: 1.009
Units: --
Reference Range: (1.009-1.025)

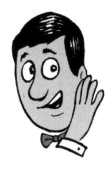

"You probably already know this, but here's a reminder.
Hypo means low, and hyper means high. How cool is that!"

The pH of a solution is a measure of the concentration of hydrogen ions. The pH scale goes from 0 to 14. Solutions with a pH between 0 and 7 are acidic, and solutions with a pH between 7 and 14 are basic. Just to give you a feel for pH values, Table F-2 gives the typical pH for several common items. The pH of urine should be between 5.0 and 9.0.

BASE
Liquid drain cleaner (pH=14)
Bleach, oven cleaner, lye (pH=13.5)
Ammonia solution (pH=10.5-11.5)
Baking soda (pH=9.5)
Seawater (pH=8)
Blood (pH=7.4)
Milk, urine, saliva (pH=6.3-6.6)
Black coffee (pH=5)
Grapefruit juice, soda, tomato juice (pH=2.5-3.5)
Lemon juice, vinegar (pH=2)
Battery acid, hydrochloric acid (pH=0)
ACID

Table F-2 pH for several common substances

Checking urine pH can be helpful in:

1. Diagnosing renal tubular acidosis.
2. Monitoring urine alkalinization to prevent precipitation of myoglobin in rhabdomyolysis, and to aid the elimination of certain drugs like aspirin and methotrexate.
3. Detecting different types of kidney stones.

Urine pH is highly dependant on diet, so it should always be used in conjunction with other labs.

Test Name: URINE PH
Result: 6.0
Units: --
Reference Range: (5.0-9.0)

F.2.3 Glucose

Glucose in the urine is referred to as glycosuria. There are only a few conditions that can lead to glucose in the urine.

1. Hyperglycemia.
2. Proximal tubule dysfunction (Fanconi syndrome).

Test Name: URINE GLUCOSE
Result: Neg
Units: --
Reference Range: (Neg)

F.2.4 Heme (Blood)

The urine dipstick is highly sensitive for hemoglobin, but it also detects myoglobin. Blood in the urine is not a good thing. It can be caused by:

1. Bleeding in the urinary tract from a urinary tract infection (UTI), kidney stones, genitourinary (GU) malignancy.
2. Rhabdomyolysis (acute muscle breakdown).

Test Name: URINE BLOOD
Result: Neg
Units: --
Reference Range: (Neg)

F.2.5 Protein

The dipstick test for protein is most sensitive for albumin, and not very sensitive for other proteins. Also, it is dependent on urine concentration, so the more concentrated the urine, the more sensitive the test will be. Protein in the urine can be caused by:

1. Diabetic nephropathy
2. Multiple myeloma
3. Rhabdomyolysis
4. Intravascular hemolysis
5. UTI

Test Name: UA PROTEIN
Result: 2+
Units: --

Reference Range: (Neg)

F.2.6 Leukocyte Esterase and Nitrites

These two tests should be considered together. They are used to aid in the diagnosis of UTIs.

Leukocyte esterase is an enzyme released by white blood cells (leukocytes are one of the five different types of white blood cells) and is used as a measure of white blood cells in the urinary tract. Why would there be white blood cells there? UTI, of course. This is your immune system in action.

You might be wondering why this test isn't just called "leukocytes" (as it is in some home testing kits) instead of "leukocyte esterase". Well, that's because it doesn't measure leukocyte concentration directly; it just infers their presence by the enzyme activity related to them. See the difference?

The nitrites test detects the presents of bacteria from the enterobacteriacae family, which converts the normally present nitrates found in urine to nitrites.

Test Name: LEUKOCYTE ESTERASE
Result: Neg
Units: --
Reference Range: (Neg)

Test Name: URINE NITRITE
Result: NEG
Units: --
Reference Range: (Neg)

F.2.7 Ketones

Ketones in the urine can be caused by:

1. Diabetes
2. Alcoholism
3. Starvation

Test Name: URINE KETONES
Result: Neg
Units: --
Reference Range: (Neg)

F.2.8 Bilirubin and Urobilinogen

The biochemical processes involved in the liver, kidneys, and gut to produce bilirubin and urobilinogen are quite complicated, but testing positive for these two substances may indicate liver disease. The dipstick test for bilirubin and urobilinogen has limited usefulness, and some hospitals don't even report these results.

Test Name: URINE BILIRUBIN
Result: Neg
Units: --
Reference Range: (Neg)

Test Name: UROBILINOGEN
Result: Neg
Units: EU/dl
Reference Range: (<1.0)

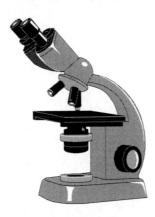

For urine microscopy, a lab technician will examine the urine sample under a microscope to quantify:

1. White blood cells
2. Red blood cells
3. Bacteria
4. Crystals
5. Casts

F.3.1 Red Blood Cells (RBCs)

Red blood cells are reported as the number observed in a high-powered field (HPF) of 400x magnification. Three or more RBCs per high-powered field is considered to be abnormal. The presence of dysmorphic RBCs strongly suggests glomerular disease.

Many conditions can cause RBCs in the urine including:

1. UTI
2. Renal stone
3. GU malignancy
4. Recent instrumentation (including Foley placement)
5. Coagulopathy
6. Sickle cell anemia
7. Renal tuberculosis
8. Vigorous exercise
9. Contamination with menstrual blood

Test Name: UA - RBC/HPF
Result: 0-3
Units: /HPF
Reference Range: (0-3)

F.3.2 White Blood Cells (WBCs)

White blood cells are also reported as the number observed in a high-powered (HPF). Five or more WBCs per HPF is considered to be abnormal. Causes of WBCs in the urine include:

1. UTI
2. Indwelling urinary catheter
3. Urologic malignancy
4. Chronic interstitial nephritis
5. Interstitial cystitis
6. Intra-abdominal inflammatory process adjacent to the GU tract
7. Contamination with vaginal secretions

Test Name: UA - WBC/HPF

Result: 0-5
Units: /HPF
Reference Range: (0-5)

F.3.3 Bacteria

Bacteria are a common finding in urine microscopy and are typically caused by a UTI.

F.3.4 Crystals

Crystals are highly organized, microscopic solids usually composed of a very small number of different ions or molecules. Formation of crystals depends on the concentration of ions and molecules as well as the urine pH. Crystals in the urine are very common and usually nothing to be concerned about.

The six most common types of crystals are:

1. Uric acid crystals are most well known as the cause of gout when they form in the joints. When found in the urine they are most associated with tumor lysis syndrome caused by rapid cell death due to chemotherapy.
2. Calcium phosphate crystals. In huge quantities, calcium phosphate can lead to renal stones, but microscopic calcium phosphate crystals in the urine typically don't suggest any specific health issues.
3. Magnesium ammonium phosphate crystals are seen in UTIs with urease-producing organisms.
4. Calcium oxalate dihydrate crystals may indicate the presence of kidney stones.

5. Calcium oxalate monohydrate crystals usually are not associated with any disease, but may suggest ethylene glycol ingestion.
6. Cystine crystals are associated with cystinuria.

F.3.5 Casts

Casts are long, cylindrical structures formed in the renal tubules due to precipitation of Tamm-Horsfall protein. Their formation is promoted by acidic or concentrated urine.

There are several varieties of casts including:

1. Hyaline casts are the most common casts seen in urine. These are not specific to any disease state, but can indicate dehydration.
2. Muddy brown casts strongly suggest acute tubular necrosis (ATN).
3. Waxy casts are non-specific and are seen in a variety of renal diseases.
4. Fatty casts contain yellow/tan fat globules, and strongly suggest nephrotic syndrome.
5. Pigment casts contain one of several pigment compounds such as heme or bilirubin.
6. Granular casts are believed to be from the degeneration of cellular casts.
7. Red blood cell casts are strongly suggestive of glomerulonephritis.
8. White blood cell casts are strongly suggestive of interstitial inflammation.

F.4 Summary

Table F-3 summarizes the most common UA abnormalities.

	Appearance	Specific Gravity	Protein	Leukocyte Esterase	Nitrites	RBCs	WBCs
UTI	Cloudy	Any	+/-	+	+/-	+/-	+
Dehydration	Dark Yellow	Relatively High	+/-	-	-	-	-
ATN	Dark Yellow or Amber	Relatively Low	+/-	+/-	-	+/-	+/-
Nephrotic Syndrome	Foamy	Relatively High	Severely High	-	-	-	-
Nephritic Syndrome	Red or Brown	Relatively High	Moderately Elevated	+/-	-	+	+/-

Table F-3 UA Abnormalities

Appendix G: Health Quiz

Here's a fun little 25-question quiz that summarizes some of the key points from this book. In parentheses after each question is the page where you can find the answer. If you get them all right without looking up the answers, you're a genius!

1. What are some good plant sources of protein? (p.93)

2. What is A1C and how does it differ from the standard glucose test? At what point are you considered diabetic? (p.243)

3. What does BMI stand for, and how is it computed? If you are 5'11" and weigh 186 lbs, what is your BMI? (p.215)

4. Should vegetarians supplement with vitamin B-12 or vitamin D? (p.92)

5. What does TSH stand for? Where in the body is it produced, and what is its function? (p.241)

6. Regarding thyroxin, what is the difference between T3 and T4? (p.242)

7. What does the term "whole foods" really mean? (p.97)

8. What does an elevated neutrophil count indicate? (p.230)

9. What are some good plant sources for calcium? (p.94)

10. What is the normal range for red blood cell count? What is it called when your red blood cell count is too low? (p.226)

11. What does mg/dL stand for? (p.224)

12. What are some foods that help to lower blood pressure? (p.145)

13. Are there foods that can help boost your immune system? (p.148)

14. Who are some of the health and wellness experts that you should be familiar with? (p.194)

15. When considering purchasing a prepackaged food, what is the first thing you should look for on the package? (p.97)

16. What foods help to lower cholesterol? (p.147)

17. What does eGFR stand for, and what eGFR level puts you in the category of Stage III kidney failure? (p.237)

18. What foods help to reduce inflammation? (p.150)

19. What would cause red blood cells to show up in the urine? (p.262)

20. What are the "dirty dozen" and the "clean fifteen"? (p.106)

21. What are the health benefits of regular exercise? (p.183)

22. What is the difference between "conventional" and "organic" produce? (p.104)

23. Are there plant foods that provide "good" fat? (p.133)

24. What are some keys for effective motivation? (p.24)

25. What does SAD stand for, and why is it important? (p.88)

Meet the Author

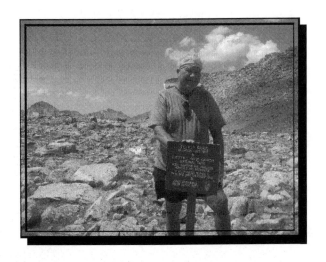

Rick holds degrees in both Mathematics and Electrical Engineering. He worked as an engineer designing microprocessor based products, teaching clients, and installing communication networks.

He now lives in beautiful Prescott, Arizona. Since retiring he has been spending time pursuing his passion for writing, playing music and teaching. Rick is currently producing a series of books on music, nature and science.

Some of his other interests include hiking, treasure hunting, recreational mathematics, photography and experimenting with microcontrollers. For more information about Rick visit his website at:

https://www.rickmckeon.com/

Other Books by Rick McKeon

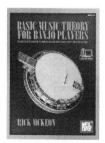

Basic Music Theory for Banjo Players: Illustrated with Playing Examples for the 5-String Banjo
ISBN: 9781513460789

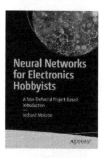

Neural Networks for the Electronics Hobbyists: A Non-Technical Project-Based Introduction
ISBN: 9781484235065

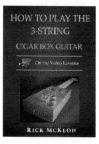

How to Play the 3-String Cigar Box Guitar: Fingerpicking the Blues
ISBN: 9781725157002

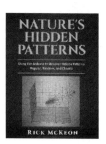

Nature's Hidden Patterns: Using the Arduino to Discover Hidden Patterns - Regular, Random, and Chaotic
ISBN: 9781719191791

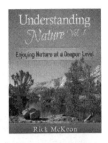

Understanding Nature Vol. 1: Enjoying Nature at a Deeper Level!
ISBN: 9341302310020

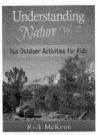

Understanding Nature Vol. 2: Fun Outdoor Activities for Kids
ISBN: 9341313333234

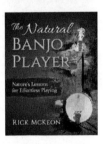

The Natural Banjo Player: Nature's Lessons for Effortless Playing
ISBN: 9341332924314

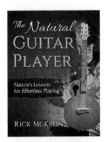

The Natural Guitar Player: Nature's Lessons for Effortless Playing
ISBN: 9341333131924

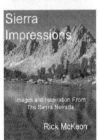

Sierra Impressions: Images and Inspiration From the Sierras
ISBN: 9341310403499

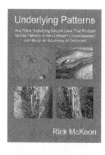

Underlying Patterns: The Search for Patterns in Nature
ISBN: 9341311343413

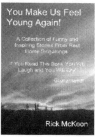

You Make Us Feel Young Again! Funny and Inspiring Stories from Entertaining at Rest Homes.
ISBN: 9341310334104

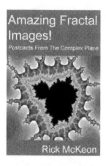

Amazing Fractal Images: Postcards From the Complex Plane
ISBN: 9341311990440

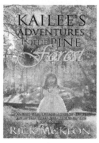

Kailee's Adventures in the Pine Forest: A Young Girl Learns Ancient Secrets from the Trees and Rocks of the Pine Forest
ISBN: 9341314293434

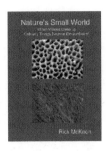

Nature's Small World: When Viewed Close up
Ordinary Things Become Extraordinary!
ISBN: 9341311943303

Index

278

Made in the USA
Lexington, KY
17 October 2019